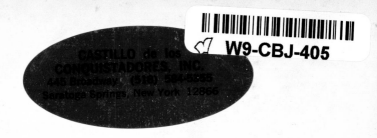

Primitive Remedies

By

John Wesley

The Renowned 18th Century
Reformer

*

How our ancestors of more than
200 years ago got well and stayed well
with simple remedies
and natural aids to good health

*

The standard home "doctor book"
in England and America for nearly 100 years
—long before the advent
of modern medicine

WOODBRIDGE PRESS PUBLISHING COMPANY
Santa Barbara, California 93111

Primitive Remedies

Published by
WOODBRIDGE PRESS PUBLISHING COMPANY
Post Office Box 6189
Santa Barbara, California 93111

Library of Congress Catalog Card Number: 73-77410

International Standard Book Number: 0-912800-29-1

Published Simultaneously in Canada

PRINTED IN THE UNITED STATES OF AMERICA
2

Contents

Page

Photographs   4
Introduction   5
Some Explanatory Notes   7
John Wesley's Own Preface   9
John Wesley's Instructions
    for Using Primitive Remedies 17
John Wesley's "Plain and Easy Rules"
    for Maintaining Good Health 19

THE PRIMITIVE REMEDIES

   "An Easy and Natural Method of
     Curing Most Diseases" 23
   (Various ailments listed, with treatments, generally in
   alphabetical order. Wesley usually indicates a preferred
   treatment with an asterisk—*—and often indicates that he
   has personally "Tried" a suggested remedy.)

John Wesley's Medicines and Their Preparation 134

SPECIAL NOTE: This authentic reproduction of John Wesley's
   Primitive Remedies is presented as a work of cultural and
   entertainment interest only. Wesley's philosophy of natural
   good health certainly provides a valid basis for preventive
   health care and many of these suggested remedies are as valid
   today as they were two hundred years ago. Nevertheless, the
   reader should consider them in the light of contemporary
   health knowledge and confer with his physician or other health
   counsellor in using them.

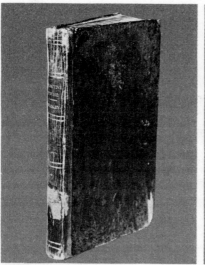
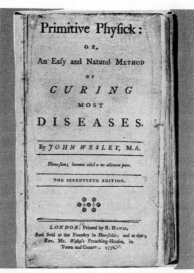

Primitive Physick:

OR,

An Easy and Natural METHOD

OF

CURING

MOST

DISEASES.

By *JOHN WESLEY*, M.A.

Homo sum; humani nihil a me alienum puto.

THE SEVENTEETH EDITION.

LONDON: Printed by R. Hawes,
And Sold at the Foundry in Moorfields; and at the
Rev. Mr. Wesley's Preaching-Houses, in
Town and Country. 1776.

(106)

189. *Inflammation or Swelling of the Scrotum.*

615. Wash it thrice a day with strong Decoction of *Agrimony.*

190. *A Scorbutic Atrophy.†*

616. Use *cold Bathing:*—Which also cures all

191. *Scorbutic Pains.*

192. *Scorbutic Sores.*

617. Put half a pound of fresh shaved *Lignum Guaiacum,* and half an ounce of *Sena* into an earthen pot that holds six quarts. Add five quarts of soft water and lute the pot close. Set this in a kettle of cold water, and put it over a fire, till it has boiled three hours. Let it stand in the kettle till cold. When it has stood one night, drink daily half a pint, new Milk-warm, fasting, and at four in the afternoon. Wash with a little of it. In three months all the Sores will be dried up. Tried.

193. *The Scurvy.‡*

618. Live

† Such a Degree of Scurvy as causes the Flesh to waste away like a *Consumption.*

‡ The *Scurvy* is known by Heaviness of Body, Weariness, Rottenness of Gums, and yellow, lead, or violet-coloured Spots on the Legs.

N.B. A *Scurvy* attended with *Costiveness,* (which is most common) is termed a *Hot-Scurvy:* One attended with *Looseness,* a *Cold-Scurvy.*

(107)

618. Live on *Turnips* for a month:

619. Or, take *Tar-Water,* morning and evening, for three months:

620. Or, Decoction of great *Water-Dock.* ☞ Perhaps there is not in Nature a more effectual plant for the Scurvy than *Water-Dock:* Especially when it appears in cutaneous eruptions. But sometimes it requires patience.——The best way of making the Decoction is this: Put half a pound of the Bark from the Root in an earthen vessel. Pour on it six pints of rain water, and boil it gently till a quart is wasted. Then keep it in a cool place for use. You may drink half a pint warm, two, three, or four times a day.

It cures also, Relaxation, or Wind at the Stomach, and all disorders proceeding therefrom.——It cures all diseases of the Nerves, as Twitchings, Contractions, Tremblings, Convulsions, Palsies, febrile Heats and Colds, Head-achs, Vertigos, Vapours, Melancholy.

621. Or, three spoonfuls of *Nettle-juice* every morning: Tried.

622. Or, Decoction of *Burdock.* Boil three ounces of the dried Root in two quarts of water to three pints. Take half a pint daily; unless it purges too much, if so take less. A Decoction of the Leaves (boiling one leaf four minutes in a quart of water) has the same Effect.

623. Or, take (from the small Branches in Spring,—from the branching roots in Autumn) four ounces of the fresh inner *Elm-Bark:* Boil them in two quarts of water to three pints,

E6

and

One of many editions of John Wesley's book, Primitive Physick—or Primitive Remedies—in the eighteenth century. Above, left: the leather-bound original; above, right: the title page; below: a typical opening showing the original, now archaic type style.

Introduction:

A Great Reformer's Amazing "Doctor Book"

How did your great-great grandparents get well and stay well—two hundred years ago?

It was an age when most health practices were derived from hearsay, folklore, and superstition—even those of many physicians.

In this setting, one of the first systematic books for the people on how to attain good health and how to treat disease was prepared by none other than John Wesley, the famous reformer, evangelist, and founder of the Methodist church.

Wesley's concern was for the common people and it was his purpose to give them "a plain and easy way of curing most diseases"; "to set down cheap, safe, and easy medicines; easy to be known, easy to be procured, and easy to be applied by plain, unlettered men." In uncommon or persistent cases, he advised "every man without delay to apply to a Physician that fears God."

Wesley called this work PRIMITIVE PHYSICK, which in the language of the day meant, more or less, "Basic Medical Care."

It is not strange that Wesley, a clergyman, should attempt what no physician had accomplished in compiling so concise and practical a guide for laymen. Medical knowledge of the day was so sparse that it could easily be included in any gentleman's education. Many men, now better known in other fields, were also, in fact, physicians.

Moreover, Wesley—though an Oxford man and deeply interested in science—was firmly opposed to many of the methods practiced by some physicians of the time; particularly the use of poisonous drugs. He was a firm believer in the virtues of simple, natural remedies and the importance of maintaining good basic health.

Some of his suggested remedies seem indeed primitive today, some humorous; but many are practical and based on principles recognized by contemporary healers.

Wesley's book made a profound impression on all classes of people in its time and did much to stem the tide of misery caused by some harmful medical procedures widely used then and—alas—now.

Usually, his book offers four specific remedies for each of nearly three hundred ailments. In some instances, Wesley indicated that he had personally "Tried" the suggested remedy.

We would not advise the reader to try some of the remedies without the guidance of a competent physician; obviously much more is known today about some of the ailments listed.

Without fail, however, one should read Wesley's own "Preface" and his "Plain, Easy Rules" with great care for they offer an extremely important and still-valid philosophy and program of health and well-being supported by "the fear of God."

The edition reproduced here is one in which the now-archaic and hard-to-read eighteenth century type has been replaced by more modern type faces, but the words and the spirit are Wesley's own, just as he gave them freely to the people so many years ago.

—Howard B. Weeks, Ph.D.

Notes:

Understanding Some of Wesley's Terms

Section

No. 1: Decoction (a term used throughout the book)—an extract obtained by boiling herbs or other materials.

No. 6: St. Anthony's fire—erysipelas.

No. 7: Glyster—an enema.

No. 10: Issue—a suppurating sore kept open by inserting an irritant, such as a small piece of wood.

No. 25: Goulard's extract of lead—extract of Saturn. (From an old medical book: Take 1 lb. Letharge, 2 pints of vinegar made of French wine. Put together in a glazed earthen pipkin and simmer for an hour and a quarter, stirring the while with a wooden spatula. After allowing to settle, pour off the liquor on top into bottles for use.)

No. 26: Brimstone—should read quicksilver.

No. 55: Costiveness—constipation.

No. 65: Hungary water—a distilled water containing aromatic oils from the tops of flowers of Rosemary or other materials.

No. 73: Bristol water—a lukewarm water containing sulphur and iron, occuring naturally.

No. 86: Gutta serena—blindness, especially with no readily apparent cause.

No. 88: Lunar caustic—silver nitrate.

No. 101: The fallling sickness—epilepsy.

No. 102: Falling of the fundament—a protrusion of part of the rectum.

No. 103 (also 115, 121): Elixir of vitriol—see No. 46.

No. 112: Fistula—a narrow duct such as may be formed from an abcess to the surface. Special note: in another edition Wesley cautions against the use of the mercury sublimate preparation. He also offers an antidote in Section No. 177.

No. 117: Aqua vitae—brandy.
No. 139: Iliac (ileac) passion—a bowel obstruction.
No. 142: The King's Evil—scrofula, a tubercular-like illness with lymphatic swelling and inflamation of the joints.
No. 156: Dragon's blood—a resin.
No. 162: Nettle rash—also prickly heat.
No. 205: Manna—an exudate from Fraxinus ornus. Ichorose—a thin fluid from a sore.
No. 212: Crab verjuice—acid liquid from crab apples.
No. 223: Carduus Benedictus—blessed thistle.
No. 226: Raging fit—Wesley refers to great pain caused by the passing of a stone. (See No. 225.)
No. 230: Stranguary—slow and painful urination.
No. 246: "Children using coral"—as a device to chew on during teething.
No. 283: Alterative—a dosage of medicine that affects the disease in some way but does not cure it.

Here is Wesley's explanation for some omissions in this edition of Primitive Remedies:

"It is because they are not safe, but extremely dangerous that I have omitted (together with antimony) ... opium, the bark (Peruvian), steel, and most preparations of quicksilver (except in a very few cases). ...Far too strong for common men to grapple with. ...

"In uncommon or complicated cases ... I again advise every man without delay to apply to a Physician that fears God."

—John Wesley, 1755.

8

PREFACE.

WHEN man came first out of the hands of the Great Creator, clothed in body, as well as in soul, with immortality and incorruption, there was no place for physic, or the art of healing. As he knew no sin, so he knew no pain, no sickness, weakness, or bodily disorder. The habitation wherein the angelic mind, the Divine Particulæ Auræ, abode, although originally formed of the dust of the earth, was liable to no decay. It had no seeds of corruption or dissolution within itself; and there was nothing without to injure it ; heaven and earth, and all the host of them were mild, benign, and friendly to human nature. The entire creation was at peace with man, so long as man was at peace with his Creator. So that well might the morning stars sing together, and all the sons of God shout for joy.

2. But since man rebelled against the Sovereign of heaven and earth, how entirely is the scene changed? The incorruptible frame hath put on corruption, the immortal hath put on mortality. The seeds of wickedness and pain, of sickness and death, are now lodged in our inmost substance; whence a thousand disorders continually spring, even without the aid of external violence. And how is the number of these increased by every thing round about us? The heavens, the earth, and all things contained therein, conspire to punish the rebels

against their Creator. The sun and moon shed unwholsome
influences from above ; the earth exhales poisonous damps
from beneath ; the beasts of the field, the birds of the air,
the fishes of the sea, are in a state of hostility ; the air itself
that surrounds us on every side, is replete with shafts of
death ; yea, the food we eat daily saps the foundation of
that life which cannot be sustained without it. So has the
Lord of All secured the execution of His decree—"Dust
thou art, and unto dust shalt thou return."

3. But can nothing be found to lessen those inconvenien-
ces which cannot be wholly removed? To soften the evils
of life, and prevent in part the sickness and pain to which
we are continually exposed? Without question there may
One grand preventative of pain and sickness of various
kinds, seems intimated by the grand Author of Nature in
the very sentence that entails death upon us,—" In the sweat
of thy face shalt thou eat bread, till thou return to the
ground. The power of exercise, both to preserve and restore health, is greater than can well be conceived ; especially in those who add temperance thereto, who, if they do
not confine themselves altogether to eat either " Bread or
the herb of the field," (which God does not require them to
do) yet steadily observe both that kind and measure of food
which experience shows to be most friendly to health and
strength.

4. It is probable Physic, as well as Religion, was in the first
ages chiefly traditional ; every father delivering down to his
sons what he had in like manner received, concerning the
manner of healing both outward hurts and the diseases incident to each climate, and the medicines which were of the

greatest efficacy for the cure of each disorder. It is certain this is the method wherein the art of healing is preserved among the American Indians to this day. Their diseases indeed are exceeding few ; nor do they often occur, by reason of their continual exercise, and (till of late) universal temperance. But if any are sick, or bit by a serpent, or torn by a wild beast, the fathers immediately tell their children what remedy to apply. And it is rare that the patient suffers long ; those medicines being quick, as well as generally infallible·

5. Hence it was, perhaps, that the ancients, not only of Greece and Rome, but even of barbarous nations, usually assigned physic a divine original. And indeed it was a natural thought, that He who had taught it to the very beasts and birds, the Cretan Stag, the Egyptian Ibis, could not be wanting to teach man.

Sanctius his Animal, *mentisque capacius altæ.*

Yea, sometimes even by those meaner creatures, for it is easy to infer, " If this will heal that creature, whose flesh is nearly of the same texture with mine, then in a parallel case it will heal me." The trial was made—the cure was wrought—and experience and physic grew up together.

6. And has not the Author of Nature taught us the use of many other medicines by what is vulgarly termed accident ? Thus, one walking some years since in a grove of pines, at a time when many in the neighboring towns were afflicted with a kind of new distemper—little sores in the inside of the mouth —a drop of the natural gum fell from one of the trees on a book which he was reading. This he took up, and thoughtlessly applied to one of those sore places. Finding the pain immediately cease, he applied it to another, which was also

presently healed. The same remedy he afterwards imparted
to others, and it did not fail to heal any that applied it. And
doubtless numberless remedies have been thus casually discovered in every age and nation.

7. Thus far physic was wholly founded on experiment.
The European, as well as the American said to his neighbor,
" Are you sick ?   Drink the juice of this herb and your sickness will be at an end.   Are you in a burning heat?   Leap
into that river and then sweat till you are well.   Has the
snake bitten you ?   Chew and apply that root, and the poison will not hurt you."   Thus, ancient men, having a little
experience joined with common sense and common hu-
manity, cured both themselves and neighbors of most of the
distempers to which every nation was subject.

8. But in process of time, men of a philosophical turn
were not satisfied with this.   They began to enquire how
they might account for these things ?   How such medicines
wrought such effects?   They examined the human body
and all its parts ; the nature of the flesh, veins, arteries,
nerves ; the structure of the brain, heart, lungs, stomach,
bowels ; with the springs of the several kinds of animal
functions.   They explored the several kinds of animal and
mineral, as well as vegetable substances ; and hence the
whole order of physic, which had obtained to that time,
became inverted.   Men of learning began to set experience
aside—to build physic upon hypothesis—to form theories of
diseases and their cure, and to substitute these in the place
of experiments.

9. As theories increased, simple medicines were more and
more disregarded and disused. till in a course of years th

greater part of them were forgotten, at least in the politer nations. In the room of these, abundance of new ones were introduced, by reasoning, speculative men ; and those more and more difficult to be applied, as being more remote from common observation. Hence, rules for the application of these, and medical books, were immensely multiplied, till at length physic became an abtruse science, quite out of the reach of ordinary men.

10. Physicians now began to be in admiration, as persons who were something more than human. And profit attended employ as well as honor ; so that they had now two weighty reasons for their keeping the bulk of mankind at a distance, that they might not pry into the mysteries of the profession. To this end, they increased those difficulties by design, which began in a manner by accident. They filled their writings with abundance of technical terms, utterly unintelligible to plain men. They affected to deliver their rules, and to reason upon them in an abstruse and philosophical manner. They represented the critical knowledge of Astronomy, Natural Philosophy, (and what not ?) Some of them insisting upon that of Astronomy, and Astrology too, as necessary previous to the understanding of the art of healing. Those who understood only how to restore the sick to health, they branded with the name of Empirics. They introduced into practice abundance of compound medicines consisting of so many ingredients, that it was scarce possible for common people to know which it was that wrought the cure ; abundance of exotics; neither the nature nor names of which their own countrymen understood ; of chemicals, such as they neither had skill, nor fortune, nor time to prepare ; yea, and of

dangerous ones, such as they could not use without hazarding life, but by the advice of a physician. And thus both their honor and gain were secured, a vast majority of mankind being utterly cut off from helping either themselves or their neighbors, or once daring to attempt it.

11. Yet there have not been wanting from time to time, some lovers of mankind, who have endeavored, even contrary to their own interest, to reduce physic to its ancient standard; who have labored to explode it out of all the hypothesis and fine-spun theories, and to make it plain intelligible thing, as it was in the beginning; having no more mystery in it than this—" Such a medicine removes such a pain." These have demonstrably shewn, that neither the knowledge of Astrology, Astronomy, Natural Philosophy, nor even Anatomy itself is absolutely necessary to the quick and effectual cure of most diseases incident to human bodies ; nor yet any chemical, or exotic, or compound medicine, but a simple plant or root duly applied. So that every man of common sense, unless in some rare case, may prescribe either to himself or neighbor ; and may be very secure from doing harm, even where he can do no good.

12. Even in the last age there was something of this kind done, particularly by the great and good Dr. Sydenham ; and in the present, by his pupil, Dr. Dover, who has pointed out simple medicines for many diseases. And some such may be found in the writings of the learned and ingenious Dr. Cheyne ; who doubtless would have communicated more to the world, but for the melancholy reason he gave one of his friends, that pressed him with some passages in his works which too much countenanced the modern practice, " O Sir,

we must do something to oblige the faculty, or they will tear us in pieces."

13. Without any regard to this, without any concern about the obliging or disobliging any man living, a mean hand has made here some little attempt towards a plain and easy way of curing most diseases. I have only consulted herein, experience, common sense, and the common interest of mankind. And supposing they can be cured this easy way, who would desire to use any other? Who would not wish to have a physician always in his house, and one that attends without fee or reward? To be able (unless in some few complicated cases) to prescribe to his family as well as himself.

14. If it be said, but what need is there of such attempt? I answer the greatest that can possibly be conceived. Is it not needful, in the highest degree, to rescue men from the jaws of destruction? From wasting their fortunes, as thousands have done, and continue to do daily? From pining away in sickness and pain, either through the ignorance or dishonor of physicians. Yea, and many times throw away their lives after their health, time, and substance.

Is it enquired, but are there not books enough already on every part of the art of medicine? Yes, too many ten times over, considering how little to the purpose the far greater part of them speak. But besides this, they are too dear for poor men to buy, and too hard for plain men to understand.

Do you say, " But there are enough of those collections of receipts." Where? I have not seen one yet, either in our own or any other tongue, which contains only safe, and cheap, and easy medicines. In all that have yet fallen into my hands, I find many dear and many far-fetched medicines ;

besides many of so dangerous a kind as a prudent man
would never meddle with.   And against the greater part of
these medicines there is a further objection—they consist of
too many ingredients.   The common method of compounding or re-compounding medicines can never be reconciled
to common sense.   Experience shews, that one thing will
cure most disorders, at least as well as twenty put together.
Then why do you add nineteen?   Only to swell the apothe-
cary's bill.   Nay, possibly, on purpose to prolong the distemper, that the doctor and he may divide the spoil.

But admitting there is some quality in the medicine pro-
posed which has need to be corrected, will not one thing
correct it as well as twenty?   It is possible, much better
And if not, there is a sufficiency of other medicines which
need no such correction.

How often, by thus compounding medicines of opposite
qualities, is the virtue of both utterly destroyed?   Nay, how
often do those joined together destroy life, which singly,
might have preserved it?   This occasioned that caution of
the great Boerhaave, against mixing things without evident
necessity, and without full proof of the effect they will produce when joined together, as well as of that they produce
when asunder ; seeing (as he observes) several things which,
separately taken, are safe and powerful medicines, when
compounded, not only lose their former powers, but com-
mence a strong and deadly poison.

PRIMITIVE REMEDIES.

————o•◦•◦•oo————

MANNER OF USING THE MEDICINES.

As to the manner of using the medicines here set down, I would advise, as soon as you know your distemper, which is very easy unless in a complication of disorders, and then you would do well to apply to a physician that fears God. For one that does not, be his fame ever so great, I should expect a curse rather than a blessing.

First.—Use the first of the remedies for that disease which occurs in the ensuing collection, unless some other of them be easier to be had, and then it may do just as well.

Secondly.—After a competent time, if it takes no effect, us the second, and the third, and so on. I have purposely set down, in most cases, several remedies for each disorder, not only because all are not equally easy to be procured at all times, and in all places, but likewise, because the medicine which cures one man will not always cure another of the same distemper. Nor will it cure the same man at all times. Therefore it was necessary to have a variety. However, I have subjoined the letter (I) to those medicines which some think are infalliable. (Tried) to those which I have found to be of the greatest efficacy.   I believe many others to be of equal virtue, but it has not laid in my way to make the trial. One I must aver from personal knowledge, grounded on a thousand experiments, to be far superior to all other medicines I have known—I mean electricity.   I cannot but entreat those who are well-wishers to mankind to make full proof of this.   Certainly it comes the nearest to a universal medicine of any yet known in the world.   Most of the medicines which I prefer to the rest are now marked with an asterisk.*

Thirdly.—Observe all the time the greatest exactness in your regimen or manner of living.   Abstain from all mixed or high-seasoned food.   Use plain diet easy of digestion, and this as sparingly as you can consistently with ease and strength.—Drink only water if it agrees with your stomach.   Use as much exercise daily in the open air as you can, without weariness.   Sup at six or seven on the lightest food ; go to bed early, and rise betimes.   To persevere with steadiness in this course, is often more than half the cure. Above all, add to the rest, for it is not labor lost, that old-fashioned medicine—*prayer ;* and have faith in God, who " Killeth and maketh alive, who bringeth down to the grave and bringeth up."

For the sake of those who desire, through the blessing of God, to retain the health which they have recovered, I have added a few plain easy rules, briefly transcribed from Dr. Cheyne.

PLAIN EASY RULES.

1. (I) The air we breathe is of great consequence to our health. Those who have been long abroad in easterly or northerly winds should drink some warm pepper tea on going to bed, or a draught of toast and water.

2. Tender people should have those who lie with them, or are much about them, sound, sweet, and healthy.

3. Every one that would preserve health should be as clean and sweet as possible in their houses, clothes, and furniture.

II. 1. The great rule of eating and drinking is to suit the quality and quantity of the food to the strength of the diges-tion; to take always such a sort and such a measure of food as sits light and easy on the stomach.

2. All pickled, or smoked, or salted food, and all high-seasoned, is unwholesome.

3. Nothing conduces more to health than abstinence and plain food, with due labor.

4. For studious persons, about eight ounces of animal food, and twelve of vegetable, in twenty-four hours, is suffi-cient.

5. Water is the wholesomest of all drinks; it quickens the the appetite and strengthens the digestion most.

6. Strong, and more especially spiritous liquors, are a cer-tain, though slow, poison.

7. Experience shows there is very seldom any danger in leaving them off all at once.

8. Strong liquors do not prevent the mischiefs of a surfeit, or carry it off so safely as water.

9. Malt liquors are extremely hurtful to tender persons.

10. Coffee and tea are extremely hurtful to persons who have weak nerves.

III. 1. Tender persons should eat very light suppers, and that two or three hours before going to bed.

2. They ought constantly to go to bed about nine, and rise at four or five.

IV. 1. A due degree of exercise is indispensably necessary to health and long life.

2 Walking is the best exercise for those who are able to bear it; riding for those who are not. The open air, when the weather is fair, contributes much to the benefit of exercise.

3. We may strengthen any weak part of the body by constant exercise. Thus the lungs may be strengthened by loud speaking, or walking up an easy ascent; the digestion and the nerves by riding; the arms and hams by strong rubbing them daily.

4. The studious ought to have stated times for exercise, at least two or three hours a day; the one-half of this before dinner, the other before going to bed.

5. They should frequently shave, and frequently wash their feet.

6. Those who read or write much, should learn to do it standing; otherwise it will impair their health.

7. The fewer clothes any one uses by day or night, the hardier he will be.

8. *Exercise, first, should be always on an empty stomach; secondly, should never be continued to weariness; thirdly, after it, we should take to cool by degrees, otherwise we shall catch cold.

9. The flesh brush is a most useful exercise, especially to strengthen any part that is weak.

10. Cold bathing is of great advantage to health; it prevents abundance of diseases. It promotes perspiration, helps the circulation of the blood, and prevents the danger of catching cold. Tender persons should pour water upon the head before they go in, and walk swiftly. To jump in with the head foremost is too great a shock to nature.

V. 1. Costiveness cannot long consist with health; therefore care should be taken to remove it at the beginning, and, when it is removed, to prevent its return by soft, cool, opening diet.

2. Obstructed perspirations (vulgarly called catching cold) is one great source of diseases. Whenever there appears the least sign of this, let it be removed by gentle sweats.

VI. 1. The passions have a greater influence upon health than most people are aware of.

2. All violent and sudden passions dispose to, or actually throw people into acute diseases.

3. Till the passion which caused the disease is calmed, medicine is applied in vain.

4. The love of God, as it is the sovereign remedy of all miseries, so in particular it effectually prevents all the bodily

---

* In malarial districts, always take a cup of coffee as soon as possible after rising from bed in the morning.

disorders the passions introduce, by keeping the passions themselves within due bounds ; and by the unspeakable joy and perfect calm serenity and tranquility it gives the mind, it becomes the most powerful of all the means of health and long life.

AN EASY AND NATURAL METHOD

OF CURING MOST DISEASES.

---

1. ABORTION, (TO PREVENT.)

Women of a weak or relaxed habit should use solid food, avoiding great quantities of tea and other weak and watery liquors. They should go soon to bed and rise early, and take frequent exercise but avoid being over-fatigued.

If of full habit, they ought to use a spare diet, and chiefly of the vegetable kind, avoiding strong liquors and everything that may tend to heat the body, or increase the quantity of blood.

In the first case, take daily half pint of decoction of Lignum Guaiacum ; boiling an ounce of it in a quart of water for five minutes.

In the latter case, give half a drachm of powdered nitre in a cup of water-gruel, every five or six hours ; in both cases she should sleep on a hard mattrass with her head low, and be kept cool and quiet.

2. FOR AN AGUE.*

Go into the cold bath just before the cold fit.

NOTHING tends more to prolong an ague than indulging a lazy, indolent disposition. The patient ought therefore, between the fits, to take as much exercise as he can bear, and to use a light diet, and, for common drink, lemonade is the most proper.

When all other means fail, give blue vitrol, from one grain to two grains in the absence of the fit, and repeat it three or four times in twenty-four hours.

Or, take a handful of groundsel, shred it small, put it into a paper bag four inches square, pricking that side which is to be next the skin full of holes ; cover this with a thin linen, and wear it on the pit of the stomach, renewing it two hours before the fit. (Tried.)

Or, apply to the stomach a large onion, slit.

Or, melt two pennyworth of frankincense, spread it on linen, grate a nutmeg upon it, cover it with linen, and hang this bag on the pit of the stomach. I have never yet known it fail.

Or, boil yarrow in new milk till it is tender enough to spread as a plaster. An hour before the cold fit apply this to the wrists, and let it be on till the hot fit is over. If another fit comes use a fresh plaster. This often cures a Quartan.

Or, drink a quart of cold water just before the cold fit, then go to bed and sweat.

---

* An ague is an intermitting fever, each fit of which is preceded by a cold shivering, and goes off in a sweat.

Or, make six middling pills of cobwebs. Take one a little before the cold fit; two a little before the next fit, (suppose the next day ;) the other three, if need be, a little before the third fit. This seldom fails.

Or, put a teaspoonful of salt of tartar into a large glass of spring water, and drink it by little and little ; repeat the same dose the next two days before the time of the fit.

Or, two small teaspoonful of sal prunella an hour before the fit. It commonly cures in thrice taking.

Or, a large spoonful of powdered camomile flowers.

Or, a tea-spoonful of spirits of hartshorn in a glass of water·

Or, eat a small lemon, rind and all.

In the hot fit, if violent, take eight or ten drops of laudanum; if costive, in hiera picra. (A preparation of aloes.)

Doctor Lind says, an ague is certainly cured by taking from ten to twenty drops of laudnum, with two drachms of syrup of poppies, in any warm liquid, half an hour after the heat begins.

It is proper to take a gentle vomit, and sometimes a purge, before you use any of these medicines. If a vomit is taken two hours before the fit is expected, it generally prevents that fit, and sometimes cures an ague, especially in children. It is also proper to repeat the medicine (whatever it be) about a week after, in order to prevent a relapse. Do not take any purge soon after. The daily use of the flesh brush, and frequent cold bathing, are of great use to prevent relapses.

Children have been frequently cured by wearing a waistcoat in which bark was quilted.*

* Peruvian Bark.

3. TERTIAN AGUE.*

Is often cured by taking a purge one day, and the next bleeding in the beginning of the fit.

Or, take a tea-spoonful of salt of tartar in spring water. This often cures double Tertians, tripple Quartans, and long lasting fevers, especially if senna be premised twice or thrice

Or, apply to each wrist a plaster of molases and soot. (Tried.)

Or, use the cold bath, unless of an advanced age or extremely weak. But when you use this on any account whatever, it is proper.

To bleed or purge before you begin.†

To go in cool ; to emerge at once but not head foremost; to stay in only two or three minutes, or less at first.

Never to bathe on a full stomach.

To bathe twice or thrice a week at least, till you have bathed nine or ten times.

To sweat immediately after it (going to bed) in palsies, rickets, and in all diseases wherein the nerves are obstructed.

You may use yourself to it without any danger, by beginning in May, and at first just plunging in, and coming out immediately ; but many have begun in winter without any inconvenience.

4. A DOUBLE TERTIAN.

Take before the fit, (after a purge or two) three ounces of cichory water, half a drachm of salt of tartar, and fifteen drops of spirit of sulphur.

---

*That is an ague which returns every other day. †Bleeding seldom used

To perfect the cure, on the fourth day after you miss the fit, take two drachms of senna, half a drachm of salt of tartar infused all night in four ounces of cichory water. Strain it and drink it.

5 A QUARTAN AGUE.*

Apply to the suture of the head, when the fit is coming, wall July flowers, beating together leaves and flowers with a little salt. Keep it on till the hot fit is over. Repeat this if need be.

Use strong exercise (as riding or walking, as far as you can bear it) an hour or two before the fit. If possible, continue it till the fit begins. This alone will frequently cure. (Tried.)

Or, apply to the wrists a plaster of turpentine ; or of bruised pepper mixed with molasses.

Or, apply oil of turpentine to the small of the back before the fit.

For a tertian or quartan, vomit with ten grains of ipeca-cuanha an hour before the cold fit begins ; then go to bed and continue a large sweat by lemonade, (that is, lemon, sugar, and water) for six or eight hours. This usually cures in three or four times. If it does not, use the cold bath between the fits.

Or, take twenty grains of powdered saffron before the fit, in a glass of white wine.

6. ST. ANTHONY'S FIRE.†

Take a glass of tar-water warm in bed every hour, wash-ing the part with the same.

---

* That is, an ague which misses two days ; coming on Monday (sup-pose) and again on Thursday.

TAR-WATER is made thus :—Put a gallon of cold water to
a quart of Norway tar, stir them together with a flat stick for
five or six minutes. After it has stood covered for three
days pour off the water clear, bottle and cork it.

Or, take a decoction of elder leaves as a sweat ; applying
to the part a cloth dipped in lime-water, mixed with a little
camphorated spirit of wine.

LIME-WATER is made thus :—"Infuse a pound of good quick-
lime in six quarts of spring water for twenty-four hours.
Decant and keep it for use."

Or, take two or three gentle purges. No acute fever bears
repeated purges better than this, especially when it affects
the head ; in the meantime boil an handful of sago, two
handful of elder leaves or bark, and an ounce of alum in
two quarts of forge water to a pint ; wash with this every
night.

If the pulse be low, and the spirits sunk, nourishing
broths and a little negus may be given to advantage.

Or, let three drachms of nitre be dissolved in as much
elder-flower tea as the patient can drink in twenty-four hours.
If the disease attacks the head, bleeding is necessary.

Dressing the inflammation with greasy ointment, or salves
etc., is very improper.

Bathing the feet and legs in warm water is serviceable,
and often relieves the patient much. In Scotland the common people cover the part with a linen cloth covered with
meal.

---

† St. Anthony's fire is a fever attended with red and painful swelling,
full of pimples, which afterwards turn into small blisters on the face or
some other part of the body. The sooner the eruption is the less danger.
Let your diet be only water-gruel, or barley broth, with roasted apples.

7. THE APOPLEXY.*

To prevent, use the cold bath, and drink only water.

In the fit, put a handful of salt into a pint of cold water, and, if possible, pour it down the throat of the patient. He will quickly come to himself; so will one who seems dead by a fall. But send for a good physician immediately.

If the fit be soon after a meal, do not bleed, but vomit.

Rub the head, feet, and hands strongly, and let two strong men carry the patient upright, backward and forward about the room.

A seton in the neck, with low diet, has often prevented a relapse.

There is a wide difference between the Sanguineous and Serous Apoplexy. The latter is often followed by a palsy; the former is distinguished by the countenance appearing florid, the face swelled or puffed, and the blood vessels, especially about the neck and temples, are turgid; the pulse beats strong; the eyes are prominent and fixed; the breathing is difficult and performed with a snorting. This invades more suddenly than the Serous Apoplexy. Use large bleeding from the arm or neck, bathe the feet in warm water; cupping on the back of the head with deep scarification. The garter should be tied very tight to lessen the motion of the blood from the lower extremities.

A scruple of nitre may be given in water every three or four hours.

When the patient is so far recovered as to be able to swallow, let him take a strong purge; but if this cannot be ef-

---

* An apoplexy is a total loss of all sense and voluntary motion, commonly attended with a strong pulse, hard breathing, and snorting.

fected, a glyster should be thrown up, with plenty of fresh butter and a large spoonful of common salt in it.

In the Serous Apoplexy, the pulse is not so strong, the countenance is less florid, and not attended with so great a difficulty of breathing. Here bleeding is not necessary, but a vomit of three grains of emetic tartar may be given, and afterwards a purge as before, and the powder of white helle-bore blown up the nose, etc.

THIS Apoplexy is generally preceded by an unusual heavi-ness, giddiness, and drowsiness.

8 CANINE APPETITE.*

"If it be without vomiting, is often cured by a small bit of bread dipped in wine, and applied to the nostrils."—*Dr. Scomberg.*

9. AN ASTHMA †

Take a pint of cold water every morning, washing the head therein immediately after, and using the cold bath once a fortnight.

Or, cut an ounce of stick liquorice into slices, steep this in a quart of water four and twenty hours and use it when you are worse than usual, as a common drink. I have known this give much ease.

Or, half a pint of tar-water twice a day.

Or, live a fortnight on boiled carrots only. It seldom fails.

---

* An insatiable desire of eating.
† An asthma is a difficulty of breathing from a disorder in the lungs In the common or moist asthma, the patient spits much.

*Or, take some quicksilver every morning, and a spoonful of aqua sulphurata, or fifteen drops of elixir of vitriol, in a large glass of spring water, at five in the evening. This has cured an inveterate asthma.

Or, take from ten to thirty drops of elixir of vitriol, in a large glass of spring water, three or four times a day.

ELIXIR OF VITRIOL is made thus : Drop gradually four ounces of strong oil of vitriol into a pint of spirits of wine or brandy ; let it stand three days, and add to it ginger, sliced, half an ounce ; Jamaica pepper, whole, one ounce. In three days more it is fit for use. But if the patient be subject to sour belchings, take the mixture for the asthmatic cough, (as Art. 57) after the elixir of vitriol.

Or, into a quart of boiling water put a tea-spoonful of balsamic æther : receive the steam into the lungs, through a fumigator, twice a day.

BALSAMIC ÆTHER is made thus : Put four ounces of spirits of wine, and one ounce of balsam of tulo, into a phial, with one ounce of æther. Keep it well corked : it will not keep above a week.

For present relief, vomit with a quart or more of warm water. The more you drink of it the better.

Do THIS whenever you find any motion to vomit ; and take care always to keep your body open.

10. A DRY OR CONVULSIVE ASTHMA.

Juice of radishes relieve much ; so does a cup of strong coffee, or garlic either raw or preserved, or in syrup.

---

* Only as a last resort.

Or, drink a pint of new milk morning and evening. This has cured an inveterate asthma.

Or, beat fine saffron small, and take eight or ten grains every night. (Tried.)

Take from three to five grains of ipecacuanha every morning, or five to ten grains every other evening. Do this, if need be, for a month or six weeks. Five grains usually vomit. In a violent fit, take a scruple instantly.

In an asthma, the best drink is apple water ; that is, boiling water poured on sliced apples.

The food should be light, and easy of digestion. Ripe fruits baked, boiled, or roasted, are very proper ; but strong liquors of all kinds, especially beer or ale, are hurtful. If any supper is taken it should be very light.

All disorders of the breast are much relieved by keeping the feet warm, and promoting perspiration. Exercise is also of very great importance, so that the patient should take as much every day as his strength will bear. Issues are found in general to be of great service.

Dr. Smith, in his Formulæ, recommends mustard whey as common drink in the moist asthma ; and a decoction of madder root to promote spitting.

THE DECOCTION is made thus : Boil an ounce of madder, and two drachms of mace, in three pints of water to two pints, then strain it, and take a tea-cupful three or four times a day. But the most efficacious medicine is the quicksilver and aqua sulphurata, (as Art. 45.)

N. B. Where the latter cannot be got, ten drops of oil of vitriol in a large glass of spring water will answer the same end. I have known many persons relieved, and some cured by taking as much jalap every morning as would lie on a sixpence.

11. TO CURE BALDNESS.

Rub the part morning and evening, with onions, till it is red, and rub it afterwards with honey.

Or, wash it with a decoction of boxwood. (Tried).

Or, electrify it daily.

12. BLEEDING OF THE NOSE. (TO PREVENT.)

Drink whey largely, every morning, and eat a quantity of raisins.

Or, dissolve two scruples of nitre in half a pint of water, and take a tea-cupful every hour.

To cure it, apply to the neck behind, and on each side, a cloth dipped in cold water.

Or, put the legs and arms in cold water.

Or, wash the temples, nose, and neck, with vinegar.

Or, keep a little roll of white paper under the tongue.

Or, snuff up vinegar and water.

Or, foment the legs and arms with it.

Or, steep a linen rag in sharp vinegar, burn and blow it up the nose with a quill.

Or, apply tenets made of soft linen dipped in cold water strongly impregnated with tincture of iron, and introduced within the nostrils quite through to their posterior apertures. This method, Mr. Hay says, never failed him.

Or, dissolve an ounce of alum powdered in a pint of vinegar ; apply a cloth dipped in this to the temples, steeping the feet in warm water.

In a violent case go into a pond or river. (Tried.)

13 BLEEDING OF A WOUND.

Make two or three tight ligatures toward the lower part of each joint : slaken them gradually.

Or, apply tops of nettles bruised.

Or, strew on it the ashes of a linen rag dipped in sharp vinegar and burned.

Or, take ripe puff balls, break them warily and save the powder : strew this on the wound and bind it on. (I) This will stop the bleeding of an amputated limb without any cautery.

Or, take of brandy two ounces; Castile soap, two drachms; potash, one drachm ; scrape the soap fine and dissolve it in the brandy, then add the potash : mix them well together and keep them close stopped in a phial. Apply a little of this warmed to a bleeding vessel, and the blood immediately congeals.

14. SPITTING OF BLOOD.

Take a tea-cupful of stewed prunes at lying down for two or three nights. (Tried.)

Or, two spoonsful of juice of nettles every morning, and a large cup of decoction of nettles at night, for a week. (Tried.)

Or, three spoonsful of sage juice in a little honey. This presently stops either spitting or vomiting blood. (Tried.)

Or, half a tea-spoonful of Barbadoes tar on a lump of loaf sugar at night. It commonly cures at once.

15. VOMITING BLOOD.

Take two spoonsful of nettle juice.

THIS also dissolves blood coagulated in the stomach. (Tried.)

Or, take as much saltpeter as will lie upon half-a-crown dissolved in a glass of cold water, two or three times a day.

16. TO DISSOLVE COAGULATED BLOOD.

Bind on the part for some hours a paste of black soap and crumbs of white bread.

Or, grated root of burdock spread on a rag : renew this twice-a-day.

17. BLISTERS.

On the feet, occasioned by walking, are cured by drawing a needleful of worsted through them ; clip it off at both ends and leave it till the skin peels off.

18. BILES.

Apply a little Venice turpentine.
Or, an equal quantity of soap and brown sugar well mixed.
Or, a plaster of honey and wheat flour.
Or, of figs.
Or, a little saffron in a white bread poultice.
'Tis proper to purge also.

19. HARD BREASTS.

Apply turnips roasted till soft, then mashed and mixed with a little oil of roses. Change this twice a day, keeping the breast very warm with flannel.

20. SORE AND SWELLED BREASTS.

*Boil a handful of camomile and as much mallows in milk and water. Foment with it between two flannels, as hot as can be borne, every twelve hours. It also dissolves any knot or swelling in any part.

21. A BRUISE.

* Immediately apply treacle spread on brown paper. (Tried.)
Or, apply a plaster of chopped parsley mixed with butter.
* Or, electrify the part. This is the quickest cure of all.

22. TO PREVENT SWELLING FROM A BRUISE.

Immediately apply a cloth, five or six times doubled, dipped in cold water, and dipped when it grows warm. (Tried)-

23. TO CURE A SWELLING FROM BRUISE.

Foment it half an hour, morning and evening, with cloths dipped in water as hot as you can bear.

24. A BURN OR SCALD.

Immediately plunge the part in cold water: keep it in an hour if not well before. Perhaps four or five hours. (Tried).

* Or, electrify it.   If this can be done presently, it totally cures the most desperate burn.

Or, if the part cannot be dipped, apply a cloth four times doubled, dipped in cold water, changing it when it grows warm.

* Or, a bruised onion.

Or, apply oil and strew on it powdered ginger.

25. A DEEP BURN OR SCALD.

Apply black varnish with a feather till it is well.

Or, inner rind of elder well mixed with fresh butter. When this is bound on with a rag, plunge the part into cold water.   This will suspend the pain till the medicine heals.

Or, mix lime-water and sweet oil to the thickness of cream, apply it with a feather several times a day.   This is the most effectual application I ever met with.

Or, put twenty-five drops of Goulard's extract of lead to half a pint of rain water ; dip linen rags in it, and apply them to the part affected.   This is particularly serviceable if the burn is near the eyes.

26. A CANCER IN THE BREAST,*

* Of thirteen years standing, was cured by frequently applying red poppy water, plaintain and rose water, mixed with honey and roses.   Afterwards, the water used alone perfected the cure.

---

* A cancer is a hard, round, uneven, painful swelling, of a blackish or leaden color, the veins round which seem ready to burst.   It comes commonly with a swelling about as big as a pea, which does not at first give much pain, nor change the color of the skin.

Use the cold bath—This has cured many—This cured Mrs. Bates, of LEICESTERSHIRE, of a cancer in her breast, a consumption, a sciatica, and rheumatism, which she had for twenty years. She bathed daily for a month, and drank only water.

A bleeding cancer was cured by drinking twice a day a quarter of a pint of the juice of clivers, or goose grass, and covering the wounds with the bruised leaves.

Another bleeding cancer was cured by the following receipt :

Take half pint of small beer. When it boils, dissolve in an ounce and a half bees' wax : then put in an ounce of hog's lard and boil them together. When it is cold pour the beer from it, and apply it spread on white leather. Renew it every other day. It brings out great blotches, which are to be washed with sal prunello dissolved in warm water.

Monsieur Le Febun advises—" Dissolve four grains of arsnic in a pint of water. *Take a spoonful of this, with a spoonful of milk, and half an ounce of syrup of poppies, every morning.

GENERALLY, where cold bathing is necessary to cure any disease, water drinking is so to prevent a relapse.

If it be not broke, apply a piece of sheet lead beat very thin, and pricked full of pin holes, for days or weeks to the breast. Purges should be added every third or fourth day.

Or, rub the whole breast morning and evening with spirits of hartshorn mixed with oil.

Or, keep it continually moist with honey.

Or take horse spurs† and dry them by the fire, till they

---

†These warts grow on the inside of the horses' fore-legs. *Half a tea-poonful at first.

will beat to powder. Sift and infuse two drachms in two quarts of ale; drink half a pint every six hours of new milk warm. It has cured many. (Tried).

Or, a poultice of wild parsnips, flowers, leaves, and stalks, changing it morning and evening; or, scraped carrots.

Or, take brimstone and aqua sulphurata. (See No. 45.) This has cured one far in advance in years. Dr. Cheyne says, a total ass-milk diet, about two quarts a day, without any other food or drink, will cure a confirmed cancer.

27. A CANCER IN ANY OTHER PART.

Apply red onions, bruised.

Or, make a plaster of roche-alum, vinegar, and honey, equal quantities, with wheat flour. Change it every twelve hours. It often cures in three or four days.

Or, stamp the flowers, leaves, and stalks of wild parsnips, and apply them as a plaster, changing it every twelve hours. It usually cures in a few days.

A cancer under the eye was cured by drinking a pint of tar-water daily, washing the same with it, and then applying a plaster of tar and mutton suet melted together. It was well in two months, though of twenty years standing.

28. A CANCER IN THE MOUTH.

Boil a few leaves of succory, plaintain, and rue, with a spoonful of honey, for a quarter of an hour. Gargle with this often in an hour. (I.)

Or, with vinegar and honey, wherein half an ounce of roche-alum is boiled.

Or, mix as much burnt alum and as much black pepper as lies on a sixpence, with an ounce of honey, and frequently touch the part.

Or, blow the ashes of scarlet cloth into the mouth or throat. It seldom fails.

29. CHILBLAINS, (TO PREVENT.)

Wear flannel socks ; or socks of chamois leather.

30. CHILBLAINS, (TO CURE.)

Apply salt and onions pounded together.

Or, a poultice of roasted onions hot. Keep it on two or three days if not cured sooner.

Wash them, if broke, with tincture of myrrh in a little water.

31. CHILDREN.

To prevent the rickets, tenderness, and weakness, dip them in cold water every morning, at least till they are nine months old.

No roller should ever be put round their bodies, nor any stays used. Instead of them, when they are put into short petticoats, put a waistcoat under their frocks.

Let them go bare-footed and bare-headed till they are three or four years old at least.

'Tis best to wean a child when seven months old. It should lie in a cradle at least a year.

No child should touch any spiritous or fermented liquors, nor any animal food, before two years old.

Their drink should be water. Tea they should never taste till ten or twelve years old. Milk, milk porridge, and water gruel, are the proper breakfasts for children.

32. CHIN-COUGH, OR HOOPING COUGH.

Use the cold bath daily.

Or, rub the feet thoroughly with hog's lard, before the fire at going to bed, and keep the child warm therein. (Tried.)

Or, rub the back at lying down with old rum. It seldom fails.

Or, give a spoonful of juice of pennyroyal, mixed with brown sugar candy, twice a day.

Or, half a pint of milk warm from the cow, with the quantity of nutmeg or conserve of roses dissolved in it every morning.

Or, dissolve a scruple of salt of tartar in a quarter of a pint of clear water; add to it ten grains of finely powdered cochineal, and sweeten it with loaf sugar.

Give a child within the year the fourth ofaspoonful of this four times a day, with a spoonful of barley-water after it. Give a child two years old, half a spoonful; a child above four years old, a spoonful. Boiled apples put into warm milk may be his chief food. This relieves in twenty-four hours, and cures in five or six days.

Or, from three to five grains of gum gamboge. It vomits and purges, and Dr. Cook says, always cures.

Or, take two grains of tartar emetic, and a half a drachm of prepared crab's claws, powdered; let them be mixed very well together.

One grain, one grain and a half, or two grains of this composition may be added to five or six grains of magnesia, and given in a small spoonful of milk and water in the forenoon, between breakfast and dinner, to a child a year old.

At night, if the fever is very high, half the former dose of this powder may be given with from five to ten grains of nitre.

In desperate cases, change of air alone has cured.

33. CHOLERA MORBUS, i. e. FLUX AND VOMITING.

Drink two or three quarts of cold water, if strong; of warm water, if weak.

Or, boil a chicken an hour in two gallons of water, and drink of this till the vomiting ceases.

Or, decoction of rice, or barley, or toasted oaten bread.

If the pain is very severe, stupe the belly with flannels dipped in spirits and water.

The third day after the cure, take ten or fifteen grains of rhubarb.

34. CHOPS IN WOMAN'S NIPPLES.

Apply balsam of sugar.

Or, apply butter and wax, which speedily heals them.

35. CHAPPED HANDS, (TO PREVENT.)

Wash them with flour of mustard.
Or, in bran and water boiled together.

(TO CURE.)

Wash with soft soap mixed with red sand. (Tried.)
Or, wash them in sugar and water. (Tried.)

36 CHAPPED LIPS.

Apply a little sal prunello.

37. A COLD.

Drink a pint of cold water lying down in bed.   (Tried.)
Or, to one spoonful of molasses in half a pint of water.
(Tried.)
Or, to one spoonful of oatmeal, and one spoonful of honey
add a piece of butter the bigness of a nutmeg : pour on,
gradually, near a pint of boiling water. Drink this lying
down in bed.

38. A COLD IN THE HEAD.

Pare very thin the yellow rind of an orange, roll it up inside out, and thrust a roll into each nostril.

39. THE CHOLIC, (IN THE FIT.)

* Drink a pint of cold water. (Tried.)

Or, a quart of warm water. (Tried.)

Or, of camomile tea.

Or, take from thirty to forty grains of yellow peel of oranges, dried and powdered, in a glass of water.

Or, take from thirty to forty drops of oil of aniseed on a lump of sugar.

Or, apply outwardly a bag of hot oats.

Or, steep the legs in hot water a quarter of an hour.

Or, take as much Daffy's Elixir as will presently purge· This relieves the most violent cholic in an hour or two· See Medicines.

40. THE DRY CHOLIC, (TO PREVENT.)

Drink ginger tea.

41. CHOLIC IN CHILDREN.

Give a scruple of powdered aniseed in their meat. (Tried.)

Or, small doses of magnesia.

Or, put one grain of emetic tartar into four table spoons-ful of water : a small tea spoonful will puke a child a week old ; a large tea spoonful is sufficient for one a month old ; and so on in proportion. Repeat the puke every day, or every other day, as the case requires.

This is, perhaps, the best medicine yet discovered for in-fants. It speedily cures inward fits, gripes, looseness, thrush, and convulsions in children. But if the child is costive, his bowels must be opened first with a little magnesia, or manna, before you give a puke.

42. BILIOUS CHOLIC.*

Drink warm lemonade : I know nothing like it.

Or, give a spoonful of sweet oil every hour. This has cured one judged to be at the point of death.

43. AN HABITUAL CHOLIC.

Wear a thin soft flannel on the part.

44. AN HYSTERIC CHOLIC.†

Mrs. Watts, by using the cold bath two and twenty times in a month, was entirely cured of an hysteric cholic, fits and convulsive motions, continual sweatings and vomiting, wandering pains in her limbs and head, with total loss of appetite.

In the fit, drink half pint of water with a little wheat flour in it, and a spoonful of vinegar.

Or, of warm lemonade.   (Tried.)

---

*This is generally attended with vomiting a greenish or frothy matter, with feverish heat, violent thirst, a bitter taste in the mouth, and little and high colored urine.

† Is attended with a violent pain about the pit of the stomach, with great sinking of the spirits and often with greenish vomitings.

Or, take twenty, thirty, or forty drops of balsam of Peru on fine sugar ; if need be, take this twice or thrice a day.

Or, in extremity, boil three ounces of burdock seed in water, which give as a clyster.

Or, twenty drops of laudanum in any proper clyster, which gives instant ease.

45. A NERVOUS CHOLIC.*

Use the cold bath daily for three or four weeks.

Or, take quicksilver and aqua sulphurata daily for a month.

46. CHOLIC FROM THE FUMES OF LEAD, OR WHITE LEAD, VERDIGREASE, ETC.†

In the fit, drink fresh melted butter, and then vomit with warm water.

To PREVENT OR CURE.—Breakfast daily on fat broth, and use oil of sweet almonds frequently and largely.

Smelters of metals, plumbers, etc., may be in a good measure preserved from the poisonous fumes that surround them, by breathing through cloth or flannel mufflers twice or thrice doubled, dipped in a solution of sea salt, or salt of tartar, and then dried. These mufflers might also be of great use in similar cases.

47. WINDY CHOLIC.

Parched peas eaten freely, have had the most happy effect when all other means have failed.

---

* A cholic with purging, some term the watery gripes.

† This some term the dry belly-ache. It often continues several days, with little urine and obstinate costiveness.

48. TO PREVENT THE ILL EFFECTS OF COLD

The moment a person gets into a house with his hands or feet chilled, let him put them into a vessel of water, as cold as can be got, and hold them there till they begin to glow. This they will do in a minute or two. This method likewise effectually prevents chilblains.

49. A CONSUMPTION.

Cold bathing has cured many deep consumptions. (Tried.)

One in a deep consumption was advised to drink nothing but water, and eat nothing but water gruel, without salt or sugar. In three months time he was perfectly well.

Take no food but new buttermilk, churned in a bottle, and white bread. I have known this successful.

Or, use as a common drink, spring water and new milk, each a quart, and sugar candy two ounces.

Or, boil two handsful of sorrel in a pint of whey, strain it, and drink a glass thrice a day. (Tried).

Or, turn a pint of skimmed milk with half a pint of small beer. Boil in this whey about twenty-five ivy leaves, and two or three sprigs of hyssop. Drink half over night, the rest in the morning. Do this, if needful, for two months daily. This has cured in a desperate case. (Tried.)

Or, take a cow heel from the tripe house ready dressed, two quarts of new milk, two ounces of hartshorn shavings two ounces of isinglass, a quarter of a pound of sugar candy, and a race of ginger. Put all these in a pot ; and set them in an oven after the bread is drawn. Let it continue there till the oven is near cᵊld ; and let the patient live on this. I have known this cure a deep consumption more than once.

Or every morning, cut a little turf of fresh earth, and laying down, breathe in the hole for a quarter of an hour. I have known a deep consumption cured thus.

" Mr. Masters, of Evesham, was so far gone in a consumption that he could not stand alone. I advised him to lose six ounces of blood every day for a fortnight, if he lived so long ; and then every third day ; then every fifth day for the same time. In three months he was well.—*Doctor Dover.* Tried.

Or, throw frankincense on burning coals, and receive the smoke daily through a proper tube into the lungs. (Tried.)

Or, take in for a quarter of an hour, morning and evening, the steam of white resin and bees' wax boiling on a hot fire shovel. This has cured one who was in the third stage of consumption.

Or, the steam of sweet spirit of vitriol dropped into warm water.

Or, take, morning and evening, a tea spoonful of white resin powdered and mixed with honey. This cured one in less than a month, who was near death.

Or, drink thrice a day two spoonsful of juice of water-cresses. This has cured a deep consumption.

In the last stage suck a healthy woman daily. This cured my father.

For diet, use milk and apples, or water gruel made with fine flour. Drink cider whey, barley water, sharpened with lemon juice or apple water.

So long as the tickling cough continues, chew well, and swallow a mouthful or two, of a biscuit or crust of bread twice a day. If you cannot swallow it spit it out. This will always shorten the fit, and would often prevent consumption.

50 CONVULSIONS.

Use the cold bath.

Or, take a tea spoonful of valerian root powdered, in a cup of water every evening.

Or, half a drachm of misselto powdered, every six hours drinking after it a draught of strong infusion thereof.

51. CONVULSIONS IN CHILDREN.

Scrape piony roots fresh digged. Apply what you have scraped off to the soles of the feet. It helps immediately. (Tried).

52. CONVULSIONS IN THE BOWELS OF CHILDREN.

Give a child a quarter old, a spoonful of the juice of *pellitory of the wall, two or three times a day; it goes through at once, but purges no more. Use the syrup if the juice cannot be had.

---

* An European plant. See dispensatory.

53 CORNS, (TO PREVENT).

Frequently wash the feet in cold water.

54 CORNS, (TO CURE.)

Apply fresh, every morning, the yeast of small beer spread on a rag.

Or, after paring them close, apply bruised ivy leaves daily, and in fifteen days they will drop out. (Tried.)

Or, apply chalk powdered and mixed with water. This also cures warts.

Some corns are cured by a pitch plaster.

All are greatly eased by steeping the feet in hot water wherein oat meal is boiled. This also helps dry and hot feet.

55. COSTIVENESS.

Rise early every morning.

Or boil in a pint and a half of broth, half a handful of mallow leaves chopped, strain this and drink it before you eat anything else. Do this frequently, if needful.

Or, breakfast twice a week or oftener, on water gruel with currants. (Tried.)

Or, take the bigness of a large nutmeg of cream of tartar mixed with honey, as often as you need.

Or, take daily, two hours before dinner a small tea cupful of stewed prunes.

Or, use for common drink, water or treacle beer, impregnated with fixed air.

Or, live upon bread made of wheat flour with all the bran in it.

Or, boil an ounce and a half tamarinds in three pints of water to a quart. In this strained, when cold, infuse all night two drachms of senna, and one drachm of red rose leaves, drink a cupful every morning.

56. A COUGH.

Every cough is a dry cough at first. As long as it continues so, it may be cured by chewing immediately after you cough, the quantity of a pepper corn of Peruvian bark. Swallow your spittle as long as it is bitter, and spit out the wood. If you cough again, do this again. It very seldom fails to cure any dry cough. I earnestly desire every one, who has any regard for his health, to try this within twenty-four hours after he perceives a cough.

Or, drink a pint of cold water lying down in bed. (Tried.)

Or, make a hole through a lemon and fill it with honey. Roast it and catch the juice. Take a tea spoonful of this frequently. (Tried.)

57. AN ASTHMATIC COUGH.

Take Spanish liquorice two ounces, salt of tartar half an ounce; boil the liquorice in three pints of water to a quart: add the salt to it when it is blood warm. Drink two spoonsful of this every two hours. It seldom fails. (Tried.) I have known this cure an inveterate moist asthma.

58. A CONSUMPTIVE COUGH.

To stop it for a time, at lying down keep a little stick liquorice shaved like horse radish, between the cheek and gums. I believe this never fails.

59. A CONVULSIVE COUGH.

Eat preserved walnuts.

60. AN INVETERATE COUGH.

Wash the head in cold water every morning.

Or, use the cold bath.   It seldom fails.

Or, peel and slice a large turnip, spread coarse sugar between the slices, and let it stand in a dish till all the juice drains down.   Take a spoonful of this when you cough.

Or, take a spoonful of syrup of horehound morning and evening. (Tried.)

Or, take from ten to twenty drops of elixir of vitriol, in a glass of water, twice or thrice a day.   This is useful when the cough is attended with costiveness, or a relaxation of the stomach and lungs.

61. A PLEURITIC COUGH.

Powder an ounce of spermaceti fine.   Work it in a mortar with the yolk of a new laid egg. Mix them in a pint of of white wine. and take a small glass every three hours.

62. A TICKLING COUGH.

Drink water whitened with oatmeal four times a day.

Or, keep a piece of barley sugar or sugar candy constantly in the mouth.

63. VIOLENT COUGHING FROM A SHARP AND THIN RHEUM.*

Work into old coserve of roses as much as you can of pure frankincense powdered as fine as possible. Take a bolus of this t wice or thrice a day.

Or, take half a grain of inspissated milky juice of sow thistle, once or twice a day. It has the anodyne and anti-spasmodic properties of opium without its narcotic effects Or it may be made into laudnum in the same manner as opium is, and five or six drops taken on a lump of sugar thrice a day.

The milky juice of all the sowthistles, dandelions, and lettuces, have nearly the same virtues.

Or, use milk diet as much as possible.

64. THE CRAMP, (TO PREVENT.)

Tie your garter smooth and tight under your knee at going to bed : it seldom fails.

Or, take a half a pint of tar water morning and evening.

Or, be electrified through the part which uses to be affect.

---

* A thin fluid secreted by the glands.

ed.   This generally prevents it for a month, sometimes for a twelvemonth.

Or, to one ounce and a half of spirits of turpentine, add flour of brimstone and sulphur vivum, of each half an ounce, smell to it at night three or four times.

Or, lay a roll of brimstone under your pillow.

65. THE CRAMP, (TO CURE.)

Strongly put out your heel.

Or, chafe the part with Hungary water.

Or, hold a roll of brimstone in your hand.   I have frequently done this with success.

66. A CUT.

Keep it closed with your thumb for a quarter of an hour, Then double a rag five or six times, dip it in cold water, and bind it on.   (Tried.)

Or, bind on toasted cheese.   This will cure a deep cut.

Or, pounded grass.   Shake it off after twelve hours, and, if need be, apply fresh.

67. DEAFNESS.

Be electrified through the ear.   (Tried.)

Or, use the cold bath.

Or, put a little salt into the ear.

Or, drop into it a tea spoonful of salt water.

Or, three or four drops of onion juice at lying down, and stoped in with a little wool,

68. DEAFNESS FROM WAX.

Syringe the ear with warm water. (Tried.)

69. DEAFNESS WITH A DRY. EAR.

Mix brandy and sweet oil; dip black wool in this and put it into the ear. When it grows dry, wash it well in brandy, dip it and put it in again.

70. DEAFNESS WITH A HEADACHE AND BUZZING IN THE HEAD.

Peel a clove of garlic, dip it in honey, and put it into your ear at night with a little black wool. Lie with that ear uppermost. Do this, if need be, eight or ten nights (Tried.)

71. A SETTLED DEAFNESS.

Take a red onion, pick out the core, and fill up the place with oil of roasted almonds. Let it stand a night then bruise and strain it. Drop three or four drops into the ear morning and evening, and stop it with black wool.

72. DELIVERY.

After delivery in child birth, the mother's milk is the only proper purge for the child. Let it begin to suck ten or twelve hours after the birth.

73. A DIABETES.‡

Drink wine, boiled in ginger, as much and as often as your strength will bear. Let your drink be milk and water. All milk meats are good.

Or, drink three or four times a day a quarter of a pint of alum posset, putting three drachms of alum to four pints of milk. It seldom fails to cure in eight or ten days.—*Dr. Mead.*

* Or, infuse half an ounce of cantharides in a pint of elixir of vitriol. Give from fifteen to thirty drops in Bristol water twice or thrice a day.

74. THE DROPSY.†

Use the cold bath daily, after purging.

Or, rub the swelled parts with salad oil by a warm hand,

---

‡ A diabetes is a frequent and large discharge of sweetish urine, attended with a constant thirst aud a wasting of the whole body.

*Use with caution.

† A dropsy is a preturnatural collection of water in the head, breast, belly, or all over the body. It is attended with a continual thirst. The part swelled pits if you press it with your fingers. The urine is pale and little.

at least one hour a day. This has done wonders in some cases.

Or, cover the whole belly with a large new sponge dipped in strong lime water, and then squeezed out. This bound on often cures, even without any sensible evacuation of water.

Or, apply green dock leaves to the joints and soles of the feet, changing them once a day.

Or, mix half an ounce of amber with a quart of wine vinegar. Heat a brick, only not red hot, and put it into a tub. Pour them upon it and hold the part swelled over the smoke, covering the tub close to keep in the smoke. The water will come out incredibly, and the patient be cured. (Tried).

Or, eat a crust of bread every morning, fasting. (Tried.)

Or, take as much as lies upon a sixpence of powdered laurel leaves, every second or third day. It works both days. (Tried.)

Or, mix a pound of the coarsest sugar with a pint of juice of pellitory of the wall, bruised in a marble mortar. Boil it as long as any scum rises. When cool, bottle and cork it. If very bad, take three spoonsful at night and two in the morning. It seldom fails. (Tried.)

Or, make tea of roots of dwarf elder. It works by urine. every twelve or fourteen minutes (that is, after each discharge) drink a tea cupful. I have known a dropsy cure by this in twelve hours time.

One was cured by taking a drachm of nitre, every morning, in a little ale.

Tar water drank twice a day has cured many, so has an

infusion of juniper berries, roasted, and made into a liquor like coffee.

Or, three spoonsful of the juice of leeks or elder leaves. (Tried.) This cured the windy dropsy.

Or, half a pint of decoction of butcher's broom, (intermixing purges twice or thrice a week.) The proper purge is ten grains of jalap with six of powdered ginger. It may be increased or lessened according to the strength of the patient.

Or, of the decoction of the tops of oak boughs. This cured an inveterate dropsy in fifteen days.

Or, take senna, cream of tartar, and jalap, half an ounce each. Mix them and take a drachm every morning in broth. It usually cures in twenty days. This is nearly the same with Dr. Ward's powder : I suppose he took it from hence. He says it seldom fails, either in the watery or windy dropsy.

Or, be electrified. This cures dropsies supposed to be incurable.

How AMAZINGLY little is yet known, even of the human body ! Have not dropsical persons been continually advised to abstain from drink as much as possible ? but how can we reconcile this with the following undeniable facts, published in the Medical Transactions.

Jane Roberts, aged twenty, was at length constrained to take her bed by a confirmed ascites and anasarca. In this desperate case she drank as much as she would, first of small beer, and when that failed, of thin milk. After awhile her skin cracked in many places, and she continued drinking and leaking till she was quite well.

A middle-aged man in the west of England, drank every day five or six quarts of cider ; and, without any other medicine, was totally cured in a few weeks of a dropsy long supposed to be incurable.

A farmer, aged seventy, in a confirmed ascites was given over for dead. Being desperate, he drank three quarts of cold water every four and twenty hours. His whole food in the meantime was sea biscuit, sometimes with a little butter For sixteen days he seemed worse. Then he discharged, for near a week, a vast quantity of water, and was soon free from his disease, which never returned.

75. DROWNED.

Rub the trunk of the body all over with salt. It frequently recovers them that seem dead.

76. THE EAR ACHE.

Rub the ear hard for a quarter of an hour.   (Tried.)
Or, be electrified.
Or, put in a roasted fig or onion, as hot as may be. (Tried.)
Or, blow the smoke of tobacco strongly into it.
But if the ear ache is caused by an inflammation of the uvula, it is cured in two or three hours by receiving into the mouth the steam of bruised hemp seed boiled in water.

77. EAR ACHE FROM COLD.

Boil rue, or rosemary, or garlic, and let the steam go into the ear through a funnel.

78. EAR ACHE FROM HEAT.

Apply cloths four times doubled and dipped in cold water changing them when warm for an half an hour.

79. EAR ACHE FROM WORMS

Drop in warm milk, which brings them out.
Or, juice of wormwood, which kills them.

80. NOISE IN THE EARS.

Drop in juice of onions.

81. HARD WAX IN THE EARS;

Is best dissolved by syringing the ears with warm water

82. EYES BLEARED.

Drop into them juice of crab apples.

83. BLOOD-SHOT EYE.

Apply linen rags dipped in cold water for two or three hours.

Or, blow in white sugar candy, finely powdered.

Or, apply boiled hyssop as a poultice. This has a wonderful efficacy.

84. A BRUISE IN THE EYE.

Apply a plaster of the concerve of roses.

85. CLOUDS FLYING BEFORE THE EYE.

Take a drachm of powdered betony every morning.
Or, be electrified.

86. BLINDNESS.

It is often cured by cold bathing.

Or, by electrifying. (Tried.) This has cured a suffusion of sixteen, and a gutta serena of twenty four years standing.

87. DULL SIGHT.

Drop in two or three drops of juice of rotten apples often.

88. FILMS.

Dry zibethum occidentale, i. e. stercus humanum, slowly ; powder it fine, and blow it into the eye twice or thrice a day.

Or, mix juice of ground-ivy with a little honey and two or three grains of bay salt. Drop it in morning and evening.

Or, touch them cautiously every day with the lunar caustic.

89. HOT OR SHARP HUMORS.

Apply a few drops of double refined sugar melted in brandy. (Tried).

Or, boil a handful of bramble leaves with a little alum in a quart of spring water, to a pint. Drop this frequently into the eye. This likewise speedily cures cancers or any sores.

Or, lay a thin slice of raw beef on the nape of the neck (Tried.)

90. EYES OR EYE LIDS INFLAMED.

Apply as a poultice, boiled, roasted, or rotten apples warm.

Or, wormwood tops with the yolk of an egg. This will hardly fail.

Or, beat up the white of an egg with two spoonsful of white rose water into a white froth. Apply this on a fine rag, changing it so that it may not grow dry till the eye or eye-lid is well. (Tried.)

Or, dissolve an ounce of fine gum arabic in two or three spoonsful of spring water; put a drop into the inner corner of the eye, from the point of a hair pencil, four or five times a day. At the same time take as much saltpeter as will lie

upon a sixpence, dissolved in a glass of water, three or four
times a day ; abstaining from all liquors as much as possible
till cured.   White bread poultices applied to the eyes in an
inflamed state, frequently occasions total blindness.

After the inflammation is subsided, if weakness still remains, dip a finger in the white copperas eye-water and rub
round the eye three or four times a day.

N. B. All acrid eye-water and powders, put into the eyes
when they are much inflamed, horribly increase both the
pain and inflammation.

91. LACHRYMAL FISTULA,*

Apply a poultice of fine leaves of rue.

Or, wash the eye morning and evening with a decoction of
quince leaves.

92. PEARL IN THE EYE.

Apply a drop of juice of calendine with a feather thrice a
day.

Or, of three-leaved grass.   It commonly cures in seven
days.

Or, dissolve a little sal ammoniac in rose water.   Keep
this three days in a copper vessel.   Drop it twice a day into
the eye.

Or, reduce separately, to the finest powder possible, an

*This disorder in the inner corner of the eye, causes the tears to flow
involuntarily.   When it is confirmed, only a surgeon can cure it.

equal weight of loaf sugar, cream of tartar, and bole armenia; mix them together, and put a little into the eye, without blowing it in, three or four times a day.

93. SORE EYES.

Drink eye-bright tea, and wash the eyes with it.

94. WHITE SPECKS IN THE EYES.

Going to bed, put a little ear-wax on the specks. This has cured many.

95. AN EXCELLENT EYE-WATER.

Put half an ounce of lapis calaminaris powdered, into half a pint of French white wine and as much white rose-water; drop a drop or two into the corner of the eye. I have known it cure total blindness.

96. ANOTHER.

Boil very lightly one spoonful of white copperas, scraped, and three spoonsful of white salt, in three pints of spring water. When cold, bottle it in large phials without straining. Take up a phial softly, and put in a drop or two in the eye morning and evening.

IT ANSWERS the intention of almost all the preceding medicines, and takes away redness or any soreness whatever; it cures pearls, rheums, and often blindness itself. But if it makes the eye smart, add more water to it.

97. ANOTHER.

Stamp and strain ground-ivy, calendine, and daisies, an equal quantity; add a little rose water and loaf sugar. Drop a drop or two at a time into the eye, and it takes away all manner of inflammation, smarting, itching, spots, webs, or any other disorder whatsoever, yea, though the sight were almost gone.

98. AN EYE-WATER,

Which was used by Sir Stephen Fox, when he was sixty years of age, and could hardly see with the help of spectacles; but hereby in some time he recovered his sight, and could read the smallest print, without spectacles, till above eighty.

Take six ounces of rectified spirits of wine, dissolve in it one drachm of camphire, then add two small handsful of dried elder flowers. In twenty-four hours after it is infused, it is ready for use. Take out a little on a tea-spoon, dip your finger in it and bathe your forehead over your eyes and each temple with it several times, morning and night, and twice more in the day constantly. Meantime dip a soft rag in dead small beer, new milk warm, and dab each eye a dozen times, gently, morning and evening.

If it is a watery humour, you may with your finger wet the

eye lids two or three times a piece ; but be sure to shut you
eyes, or it makes them smart and burn excessiveiy.   If you
have the tooth-ache, or swelled face, rub it well on the part
and it will take away the pain.   It will cure any bruise also
if used immediately.   (Tried.)

99. WEAK EYES.

Wash the head daily with cold water.   (Tried.)

100 FAINTING ON LETTING BLOOD,

Is prevented by taking before it some good broth.

101. THE FALLING SICKNESS.*

Be electrified.   (Tried.)
Or, use the cold bath for a month, daily.
Or, take a tea-spoonful of piony root, dried and grated
fine, morning and evening for three months.
Or, half a spoonful of valerian root powdered, three times
a day, in a glass of water, for three months.
Or, half a pint of tar water, morning and evening, for
three months.
Or, a glass of juice of pellitory of the wall, every morn-
ing.

---

*In the falling sickness, the patient falls to the ground either quite
stiff or convulsed all over, utterly senseless, gnashing his teeth, and
foaming at the mouth,

Or, take five or six drops of laudanumfasting, for six or seven mornings. This has cured many.

Or, use an entire milk diet for three months. It seldom fails.

In the fit, blow up the nose a little powdered ginger. Or, leaves of assarabacca powdered.

THIS is the famous Major's snuff.

Or, blow down the throat the smoke of tobacco.

* One who is subject to the falling sickness, may prevent the fit if he feels it coming, by this simple experiment : let him always carry with him a piece of metal as broad as he is able to hold between his teeth, when his jaws are stretched to the utmost. When he feels the fit approaching, let him immediately put this between his teeth so as to keep his jaws at the utmost stretch. In about a minute this will bring him quite to himself, and prevent the fit for that time.

If one put this metal between the teeth of one that is in the fit, and force them open till his jaws are at the utmost stretch, the fit will immediately go off, and the patient very soon recover.

102. THE FALLING OF THE FUNDAMENT.

Apply a cloth covered thick with brick-dust.

Or, boil a handful of red rose leaves in a quarter of a pint of red wine, dip a cloth in it, and apply it as hot as can be borne. Do this till all is used.

103. A FALLING DOWN OF THE WOMB

May be cured in the manner last mentioned.

Or, wear a pessory of cork, and take once or twice a day a tea-cupful of the decoction of the bark, with ten drops of the elixir of vitriol.

104. EXTREME FAT.

Use a total vegetable diet. I knew one who was entirely cured of this by living a year thus: she breakfasted and supped on milk and water (with bread) and dined on turnips, carrots, or other roots, drinking water.

105. A FEVER.

In the beginning of any fever, if the stomach is uneasy, vomit; if the bowels purge ; if the pulse be hard, full, or strong, bleed.*

Drink a pint or two of cold water lying down in bed ; I never knew it to do hurt.

Or, a large glass of tar-water, warm every hour.

Or, thin water gruel sweetened with honey, with one or two drachms of nitre in each quart.

THE best of all juleps in a fever is thus : Toast a large thin slice of bread, without burning ; put it hot into a pint of cold water, then set it on the fire till it is pretty hot. In a dry heat it may be given cold ; in a moist heat, warm ; the more largely the better.   (Tried.)

Or, for a change, use pippin or wood-sorrel tea ; or pippin whey, or wood-sorrel whey.

---

*We seldom advise bleeding.

(To prevent catching any infectious fever, do not breathe near the face of the sick person, neither swallow your spittle whilst in the room. Infection seizes the stomach first.)

Or, stamp a handful of leaves of woodbine, put soft water to it, and use it cold as a clyster. It often cures in an hour.

Or, smear the wrists five or six inches long with warm molasses, and cover it with brown paper.

Or, apply molasses plasters to the head and the soles of the feet, changing them every twelve hours.

Or, use Dr. Boerhaave's fever powder, viz : Eight ounces of nitre, a quarter of an ounce of camphire, half a quarter of an ounce of saffron, and eight grains of cochineal. These are to be powdered, mixed together, and kept dry in a bottle. Ten grains taken at going to bed abate feverish heat, and procure rest. Ten grains are to be taken every three or four hours for a continued fever.

106. A HIGH FEVER,

Attended with a delirium and a vigilia, has been cured by plunging into cold water; which is a safe and sure remedy* in the beginning of any fever.

Such a delirium was often cured by applying to the top of the head a molasses plaster. (Tried).

107. AN INTERMITTING FEVER.

Drink warm lemonade in the beginning of every fit; it cures in a few days. (Tried.)

---

*Only *robust* persons should use this remedy.

Or, take a tea-spoonful of oil of sulphur in a cup of balm tea, once or twice a day.

108. A FEVER WITH PAINS IN THE LIMBS.

Take twenty drops of spirit of hartshorn in a cup of water twice or thrice in twenty-four hours.
Or drink largely of cinque-foil tea.

109. A RASH FEVER.

Drink every hour a spoonful of juice of gronnd-ivy.   It often cures in twenty-four hours.   Use this decoction when you have not the juice.

110. A SLOW FEVER.

Use the cold bath for two or three weeks, daily.

111. A WORM FEVER.

Boil a handful of rue and wormwood in water ; foment the belly with the decoction, and apply the boiled herbs as a poultice ; repeat the application night and morning. This frequently brings away worms from children who will take no internal medicine, and is likewise serviceable if the fever be of the putrid kind.

112 A FISTULA.

Wash muscle shells clean, burn them to powder, sift them

fine, mix them with hog's lard, spread it on clean wash leather, and apply it. This cured one who was thought to be at the point of death.

N. B. This also cures the piles.

Or, grind an ounce of sublimate mercury in a glass pestile, as fine as possible. Put it into a glass bottle, and pour on it two quarts of pure spring water.
Cork it close, and for six days shake it well every hour. Then let it settle for twenty-four hours. Pour it off clear, filter in a glass funnel and keep it for use, close stopped.

[Should be kept out of the reach of children and labeled poison. For external use as below.—ED.]

Or, have a vessel so contrived, that you may sit with the part in cold water a quarter of an hour, every morning. I have known a gentleman of seventy cured thereby.

Or, put a large stone of unslacked lime into four quarts of water, let it stand one night ; take four ounces of roche-alum, and four ounces of white coperas, calcine them to dryness, then powder them as fine as possible : take three pints of the above water and put the powder into it and boil it for an half hour, then let it cool, and bottle it for use. Let the fistula be syringed with this often a little warm ; and apply it twice a day. Cover with a plaster of diaculum.

This water will destroy the callosity of the edges of the fistula, which otherwise would prevent its healing, and managed as above, will heal it up at the same time.

113. TO DESTROY FLEAS AND BUGS.

Cover the floor of the room with leaves of black alder

gathered while the dew hangs upon them : adhering to these
they are killed thereby.

Or, powder stavesacre and sprinkle it on the body, or on
the bed.

114. PHLEGM.

To prevent, or cure, take a spoonful of warm water first
thing in the morning.

115. FLOODING, (IN LYING IN.)

Cover the body with cloths dipped in vinegar and water
changing them as they grow warm.   Drink cooling acid
liquors.

This is a complaint which is not to be thought little of.
Sometimes a violent flooding comes on before delivery ; and
the only way to save both the mother and the child is to deliver the woman immediately, which, being done, the flooding will generally cease.   Sometimes a slight flooding comes
on some weeks before labor ; and here if the patient be
kept cool, her diet light, and small doses of nitre often repeated, (an ounce divided into thirty parts, and one given
every four hours) she will frequently go her full time and do
well; but if it should become excessive, delivery should be
effected as soon as may be.

If a flooding should come on after delivery, the patient
should be laid with her head low, kept cool, and be in all re-
spects treated as for an excessive flux of the menses. Linen
cloths which have been wrung out of vinegar and water,
should be applied to the belly, the loins, and the thighs :

These must be changed as they grow dry, may be discontinued as soon as the flooding abates. Sometimes the following mixture will be very useful, viz : Pennyroyal-water, simple cinnamon-water, and syrup of poppies, of each two ounces; acid elixir of vitriol, one drachm. Mix and take two table-spoonful every hour. But large doses of nitre given often (a scruple every hour) is generally the most efficacious. But when all other things seem to have no effect cold water dashed upon the patient's belly will stop the flooding immediately.

116. A FLUX.

Receive the smoke of turpentine cast on burning coals This cures also the bloody flux, and the falling of the fundament.

Or put a large brown toast into three quarts of water, with a drachm of cochineal, powdered, and a drachm of salt of wormwood. Drink it all in as short a time as you conveniently can.

THIS rarely fails to cure all fluxes, cholera morbus, yea and inflammation of the bowels. Tried.

Or, take a spoonsfulof plantaine seed, bruised, morning and evening, till it stops.

Or, ten grains of ipecacuanha, three mornings successively It is likewise excellent as a sodorific.

Or, boil four ounces of rasped logwood, or fresh logwood chips, in three quarts of water to two ; strain it, and drink a quarter of a pint sweetened with loaf sugar, warm, twice

a day.   It both binds and heals.   Or, take a small **tea**-cup-
ful of it every hour.

Or, boil the fat of a breast of mutton in a quart of spring
water for an hour.   This will cure the most inveterate flux.
(Tried.

117. A BLOODY FLUX.

Apply suppository of linen dipped in aqua vitæ.

Or, drink cold water as largely as possible, taking nothing
else till the flux stops.

Or, take a large apple, and at the top pick out all the
core, and fill up the place with a piece of honey-comb, the
honey being strained out ; roast the apple in embers and eat
it, and this will stop the flux immediately.

Or, grated rhubarb, as much as lies on a shilling, with half
as much of grated nutmeg, in a glass of white wine, at lying
down every other night.   (Tried.)

Or, take four drops of laudanum,and apply to the belly a
poultice of wormwood and red roses, boiled in milk.

In a dysentery, the worst of all fluxes, feed on rice, saloup,
sago, and sometimes on beef tea ; but no flesh.

To stop it, take a spoonful of suet melted over a slow fire.
Do not let blood.

A PERSON was cured in one day by feeding on rice milk,
and sitting a quarter of an hour in a shallow tub, having in
it warm water, three inches deep.

118. GANGRENE, (TO PREVENT OR STOP A BEGINNING.)

Foment continually with vinegar, in which dross of iron
(either sparks or clinkers) has been boiled.

119. THE GOUT IN THE STOMACH.

Dissolve two drachms of Venice treacle in a glass of mountain wine. After drinking it go to bed. You will be easier in two hours, and well in sixteen.—*Dr. Dover.*

Or, boil a * pugil of tansey in a quarter of a pint of mountain wine. Drink it in bed. I believe this never fails

To prevent its return, dissolve half an ounce of gumguiacum in two ounces of sal volatile. Take a tea-spoonful of this every morning in a glaas of spring water.

This helps any sharp pain in the stomach—*Dr. Boerhaave.*

N. B. I knew a gentleman who was cured many times by a large draught of cold water.

120. THE GOUT IN THE FOOT OR HAND.

Apply a raw lean beef steak. Change it once in twelve hours till cured. (Tried.)

121. THE GOUT IN ANY LIMB.†

Rub the part with warm treacle, and then bind on a flannel smeared therewith. Repeat this it need be, once in twelve hours.

---

* A pugil is as much as you can take up between your thumb and two fingers.

† Regard not them who say the gout ought not to be cured ; they mean it cannot. I know it cannot by their regular prescriptions ; but I have known it cured in many cases without any ill effects following.

THIS has cured an inveterate gout in thirty-six hours.

Or, drink a pint of strong infusion of elder buds dry or green, morning and evening. This has cured inveterate gouts.

Or, at six in the evening, undress and wrap·yourself up in blankets ; then put your legs up to the knees in water, as hot as you can bear it. As it cools, let hot water be poured in so as to keep you in a strong sweat till ten. Then go to bed well warmed, and sweat till morning. I have known this cure an inveterate gout in a person above sixty, who lived eleven years after. The very matter of the gout is frequently destroyed by a steady use of Mynsicht's elixir of vitriol.*

122. THE GRAVEL.

Eat largely of spinach.

Or, drink largely of warm water sweetened with honey.

Or, of pellitory of the wall tea so sweetened.

Or, infuse an ounce of wild parsley-seeds in a pint of white wine for twelve days. Drink a glass of it, fasting, three months. To prevent its return, breakfast for three months on agrimony tea. It entirely cured me twenty years ago, nor have I had the least symptom of it since.

123. GREEN SICKNESS.

Take a cup of decoction of lignum guiacum (commonly called lignum vitæ) morning and evening.

---

* Elixir of vitriol of the dispensatory practicaly the same.

Or, grind together into a fine powder, three ounces of the finest steel finings, and two ounces of red sugar candy. Take from a scruple to half a drachm every morning. (I.)

124. TO KILL ANIMALCULA THAT CAUSE THE GUMS TO WASTE AWAY FROM THE TEETH.

Gargle thrice a day with salt and water.

125. TO MAKE HAIR GROW.

Wash it every night with a strong decoction of rosemary. Dry it with flannel. (Tried.)

126. THE HEAD-ACHE.

Rub the head for a quarter of an hour. (Tried.)
Or, be electrified. (Tried.)
Or, apply to each temple the thin yellow rind of a lemon newly pared off.
Or, pour upon the palm ot the hand a little brandy and some zest* of lemon, and hold it to the forehead ; or a little æther.
Or, if you have catched cold, boil a handful of rosemary in a quart of water. Put this in a mug, and hold your head, covered with a napkin, over the steam as hot as you can bear it. Repeat this till the pain ceases. (Tried.)

---

* Zest is the juice of the peel squeezed out.

Or, snuff up the nose camphorated spirits of lavender.
Or, a little of horse-radish.

127. A CHRONIC HEAD-ACHE.

Keep your feet in warm water a quarter of an hour before
you go to bed, for two or three weeks.   (Tried.)
Or, wear tender hemlock leaves under the feet, changing
them daily.
Or, order a tea-cupful of cardnus tea without sugar, fast
ing, for six or seven mornings.   (Tried.)

128. HEAD-ACHE FROM HEAT

Apply to the forehead cloths dipped in cold water.

129. A NERVOUS HEAD-ACHE.

Dry and powder an ounce of marjoram and half an ounce
of assarabacca ; mix them as snuff, keeping the ears and
throat warm.   This is of great use even in a cancer ; but it
will suffice to take a small pinch every other night, lying
down in bed.

130. A VIOLENT HEAD-ACHE.

Take of white-wine vinegar and water, each three spoons-

ful, with half a spoonful of Hungary water. Apply this
twice a day to the eyelids and temples.

131. HEMICRANIA.*

Use cold bathing.

Or, apply to that part of the head shaven, a plaster that
will stick, with a hole cut in the middle of it as big as a half
penny; place over that hole the leaves of ranunculus†
bruised and very moist. It is a gentle blister.

132. STOPPAGE IN THE HEAD.

Snuff up juice of primrose, keeping the head warm.

133. THE HEART BURNING.‡

Drink a pint of cold water. (Tried.)

Or, drink slowly decoction of camomile flowers.

Or, eat four or five oysters.

Or, chew five or six pepper corns a little, then swallow
them.

Or, chew fennel or parsley, and swallow your spittle.

---

* This is a head-ache which affects but one side of the head.

† Crow-foot.

‡ A sharp gnawing pain in the orfice of the stomach.

Sometimes a vomit is needful.
Or, a piece of Spanish liqorice.

134. THE HICCUP, (TO PREVENT.)

Infuse a scruple of musk in a quart of mountain wine, and take a small glass every morning.

(TO CURE.)

Swallow a mouthful of water, stopping the mouth and ears. (Tried.)

Or, take anything that will make you sneeze.

Or, three drops of oil of cinnamon on a lump of sugar. (Tried).

Or, two or three preserved damsons.

Or, ten drops of chemical oil of amber dropped on sugar, and then mixed with a little water.

135. HOARSENESS.

Rub the soles of the feet, before the fire, with garlic and lard well beaten together, over night. The hoarseness will be gone next morning. (Tried.)

Or, take a pint of cold water lying down.

Or swallow slowly the juice of radishes.

Or, half a pint of mustard whey lying down.

Or, a tea-spoonful of conserve of roses every night. (Tried

Or, dry nettle roots in an oven ; then powder them finely,

and mix with an equal quantity of molasses. Take a tea-spoonful twice a day.

Or, boil a large handful of wheat bran in a quart of water, strain, and sweeten it with honey. Sup of it frequently.

136. HYPOCONDRIAC AND HYSTERIC DISORDERS·

Use cold bathing.

Or, take a physic nearly every morning, and ten drops of elixir of vitriol in the afternoon, in a glass of water.

131. THE JAUNDICE.

Wear leaves of calendine upon and under the feet.

Or, take a small pill of Castile soap every morning for eight or ten days. (Tried.)

Or, beat the white of an egg thin ; take it morning and evening in a glass of water. (I.)

Or, half a pint of strong decoction of nettles, or of bur-dock leaves morning and evening.

Or, boil three ounces of burdock root, in two quarts of water to three pints. Drink a tea-cupful of this evey morn-ing.

138. JAUNDICE IN CHILDREN.

Take half an ounce of fine rhubarb, powdered, mix with it

thoroughly, by long beating, two handsful of good well
cleansed currants. Of this give a tea-spoonful every morning.

139. THE ILIAC PASSION.*

Apply warm flannels soaked in spirits of wine.
Or, hold a live puppy constantly on the belly.—*Dr.
Sydenham.*
Inflammations in general are more certainly abated by
smart purging than by bleeding.

140. AN IMPOSTHUME †

Put the white of two leeks in a wet cloth, and so roast
them in ashes, but not too much. Stamp them in a mortar
with a little hog's grease. Spread it thick plaster-wise, and
apply it, changing it every hour till all the matter is come
out, which will be in three times. (I.)

141 THE ITCH.‡

Wash the parts affected with strong rum. (Tried).

---

*In this violent kind of cholic the execremets are supposed to be
thrown up by the mouth in vomiting.
† A forming abcess.
‡ This distemper is nothing bur a kind of very small lice which bur-
row under the skin ; therefore inward medicines are absolutely needless.
Is it possible any physician should be ignorant of this ?

Or, anoint them with black soap, but wash it off soon.

Or, steep a shirt half an hour in a quart of water mixed with half an ounce of powdered brimstone. Dry it slowly and wear it five or six days. Sometimes it needs repeating. (Tried.)

Or, mix powder of white hellebore with cream for three days. Anoint the joints for three mornings and evenings. It seldom fails.

Or, beat together the juice of two or three lemons, with the same quantity of oil of roses. Anoint the parts affected. It cures in two or three times using.

142. THE KING'S EVIL.*

Take as much cream of tartar as lies on a sixpence, every morning and evening.

Or, drink for six weeks half a pint of strong decoction of devil's bit. (Tried.)

Or, use the diet drink as in the article Scorbutic Sores. I have known this cure one whose breast was as full of holes as a honey-comb.

Or, set a quart of honey by the fire to melt. When it is cold strew into it a pound and a half of quick-lime beat very fine, and sifted through a hair sieve. Stir this about till it boils up of itself into a hard lump. Beat it when cold

---

*It commonly appears first by the thickness of the lips, or a stubborn humor in the eyes, then come hard swellings in the neck chiefly, then running sores.

very fine, and sift it as before. Take of t his as much as lies
on a shilling, in a glass of water, every morning an hour before breakfast, at four in the afternoon, and at going to bed

Or, make a leaf of dr.ed burdock into a pint of tea ; take
half a pint twice a day for four months. I have known this
cure hundreds.

The best purge for the king's evil is tincture of jalap,
which is made thus : Jalap, in powder, two ounces ; Geneva,
or proof spirits, one pint. Let them infuse seven days. A
tea-spoonful or two is sufflcient for a child ten ye ars old, in a
morning, fasting ; and repeated once or twice a week, so as
to keep the stomach and bowels clean, will frequently cure
the king's evil.   But all violent purges, when repeated too
often, are pernicious.*

143. LAMENESS FROM A FIXED CONTRACTION OF THE PARTS.

Beat the yolk of a new laid egg very thin, and, by a spoonful at a time, add and beat up with it three ounces of water.
Rub this gently into the parts for a few minutes three or
four times a day.

144. LEGS INFLAMED.

Apply Fuller's earth spread on brown paper.   It seldom
fails.

---

*The tincture of jalap must be taken in any agreeable liquid.

Or, bruised or boiled turnips. Purges in most cases are absolutely necessary.

145. LEGS, SORE AND RUNNINGS.

Wash them in brandy, and apply elder leaves, changing twice a day. This will dry up all the sores, though the legs were like a honey-comb. (Tried.)

But take also a purge or two every week.

Or, poultice them with spoiled apples. (Tried.)

146. LEPROSY.*

Use the cold bath.

Or, wash in the sea often and long.

Or, mix well an ounce of pomatum, a drachm of powdered brimstone, and half an ounce of sal prunello, and anoint the parts so long as there is need.

Or, add a pint of juice of houseleek, and half a pint of verjuice, to a pint and a half of whey. Drink this, in twenty-four hours. It often cures the quinsy, and swellings on the joints.

Or, drink half a pint of celery whey, morning and evening. This has cured in a most desperate case.

Or, drink for a month a decoction of burdock leaves, morning and evening. [Tried.]

---

*In this disease the skin in many parts is covered with rough, whitish, scaly pustules, and if these are rubbed off, there remains a kind of scaly scurf.

147. LETHARGY.

Snuff strong vinegar up the nose.

Or, half a pint of decoction of water cresses, morning and evening. (Tried.)

148. LICE, [TO KILL.]*

Sprinkle Spanish snuff over the head.

Or, wash it with a decoction of amaranth.†

149. FOR ONE SEEMINGLY KILLED WITH LIGHTNING, A DAMP, OR SUFFOCATED.

Plunge him immediately into cold water.

Or, blow strongly with a bellows down his throat. This may recover a person seemingly drowned. It is still better if a strong man blows into his mouth. See the directions published by the Humane Society.

150. LUES VENEREA.

Take a little quicksilver every morning, and a spoonful of aqua sulphurata in a glass of water, at five in the afternoon. I have known a person cured by this when supposed

---

*Should be used with care.
†Prince-feather.

to be at the point of death, who had been infected by a foul nurse before she was a year old.

I INSERT this for the sake of such innocent sufferers.

151. LUNACY.

Give decoction of agrimony four times a day.

Or, rub the head several times a day with vinegar in which ground-ivy leaves have been infused.

Or, take daily an ounce of distilled vinegar.

Or, boil the juice of ground-ivy with sweet oil and white wine into an ointment. Shave the head, anoint it therewith, and chafe it every other day for three weeks. Bruise also the leaves and bind them on the head, and give three spoonsful of the juice, warm, every morning.

THIS generally cures melancholy.

The juice alone taken twice a day will cure.

Or, be electrified. (Tried.)

152. RAGING MADNESS.*

Apply to the head cloths dipped in cold water.

Or, set the patient with his head under a great water-fall

---

* It is a sure rule that all madmen are cowards, and may be conquered by binding only, without beating.—*Dr. Mead*. He also observes, that blistering the head does more harm than good. Keep the head close shaved, and frequently wash it with vinegar.

† If this is really a nervous disorder, what wonder if it should be cured by cold bathing.

as long as his strength will bear, or pour cold water on his head out of a tea-kettle.

Or, let him eat nothing but apples for a month.

Or, nothing but bread and milk. (Tried.)

153. BITE OF A MAD DOG.

Plunge into cold water daily for twenty days, and keep as long under it as possible. This has cured even after the hydrophobia was begun. †

Or, mix ashes of trefoil with hog's lard, and anoint the part as soon as possible. Repeat it twice or thrice at six hours distance. This has cured many, and particularly a dog bit on the nose by a mad dog.

Or, mix a pound of salt with a quart of water. Squeeze, bathe, and wash the wound with this for an hour ; then bind some salt upon it for twelve hours.

N. B. The author of this receipt was bit six times by mad dogs, and always cured himself by this means.

Or, mix powdered liver-wort, four drachms : black pepper, two drachms. Divide this into four parts, and take one in warm milk for four mornings, fasting. Dr. Mead affirms he never knew this fail : but it has sometimes failed.

Or, take two or three spoonsful of the juice of rib-wort, morning and evening, as soon as possible after the bite. Repeat this for two or three changes of the moon. It has not been known to fail.

IMMEDIATELY consult an honest physician.

154. THE MEASLES.†

Drink only thin water-gruel, or milk and water the more the better ; or toast and water.

If the cough be very troublesome, take frequently a spoon-ful of barley water sweetened with oil of sweet almonds newly drawn, mixed with syrup of maiden hair.

After the measles, take three or four purges, and for some weeks take care of catching cold ; use light diet, and drink barley water instead of malt drink.

155. MENSES OBSTRUCTED

Be electrified. (Tried).

Or, take half a pint of strong decoction of pennyroyal every night at going to bed.

Or, boil five large heads of hemp in a pint of water to half. Strain it and drink it going to bed, two or three nights. It seldom fails. (Tried.)

Or, take six or twelve grains of calomel, in a pill, for two or three nights. taking care not to catch cold. It vomits and purges. (Tried.)

Or, pour twelve ounces of rectified spirits of wine on four ounces of roots of black hellebore, and let it stand in a

---

* This distemper is always preceded by a violent cough, often fourteen days before the red spots come out.

warm place twenty-four hours. Pour it off, and take from
thirty to forty drops in any liquid, fasting.

It is good likewise in the green sickness, in all hypochon-
driacalcases, and in obstinate madness.

Or, burn a little sulphur of antimony on a chafing dish of
coals, and receive the smoke by a funnel. In a few minutes
it will take effect.

LET any of these medicines be used at the regular time,
as near as can be judged.

156. MENSES NIMII.

Drink nothing but cold water with a spoonful of fine flour
stirred in it. At that time drink a glass of the coldest water
you can get, and apply a thick cloth dipped in cold water.

Or, put the feet into cold water.

Or, apply a sponge dipped in red wine and vinegar.

Or, bleed in the arm. Stop the orfice often with your
finger, and then let it bleed again.

Or, boil four or five leaves of the red hollyhock in a pint
of milk, with a small qantity of sugar. Drink this in the
morning : if the person can afford it, she may add a tea-
spo uful of Balm of Gilead. This does not often fail.

* Or, reduce to a fine powder, half an ounce of alum with
a quarter of an ounce of dragon's blood. In a violent case
take a quarter of a drachm every half hour. It scarcely
ever fails to stop the flux, before half an ounce is taken.

This also cures the whites.

157. TO RESOLVE COAGULATED MILK.

Cover the woman with a table cloth, and hold a pan of hot water just under her breast, then stroke it three or four minutes. Do this twiee a day till it is cured.

158. TO INCREASE MILK.

Drink a pint of water going to bed.
Or, drink largely of pottage made with lentils.

159. TO MAKE MILK AGREE WITH THE STOMACH.

If it lie heavy, put a little salt in it ; if it curdle, sugar. For billious persons mix it with water.

160. MORTIFICATION, (TO STOP.)

Apply a poultice of flour, honey and water, with a little yeast.

161. NERVOUS DISORDERS.

When the nerves perform the office too languidly a good air is the first requisite. The patient should rise early, and, as soon as the dew is off the ground, walk ; let his breakfast be mother of thyme tea, gathered in June, using half as much as we do of common tea. Or, the common garden thyme, if the former cannot be procured. When the nerves are too sensible, let the person breathe a proper air. Let him eat veal, chickens, or mutton. Vegetables should be eat sparingly ; the most innocent is the French bean, and the best root the turnip. Wine should be avoided carefully ; so should all sauces. Sometimes he may breakfast upon a quarter of an ounce of valerian root infused in hot water, to which he may add cream and sugar. Tea is not proper. When the person finds an uncommon oppression, let him take a large spoonful of tincture valerian root.

This tincture is made thus : Cut in pieces six ounces of valerian root, gathered in June and fresh dried. Bruise it by ʰᵛ a few strokes in a mortar, that the pieces may be split, but it should not be beat into powder : put this into a quart of strong white wine ; cork the bottle and let it stand three weeks, shaking it every day ; then press it out and filter the tincture through paper.

N. B. The true wild valerian has no bad smell ; if it has, cats have urined upon it, which they will do if they can come at it.

But I AM FIRMLY PERSUADED there is no remedy in nature for nervous disorders of every kind, comparable to the proper and constant use of the electrical machine.

162 NETTLE RASH.*

Rub the parts strongly with parsley. Internals profit nothing.

---

*A slight fever attended itching, smarting, and eruption, over the body

163. OLD AGE.

Take tar-water morning and evening. (Tried.)

Or, decoction of nettles; either of these will probably renew their strength for some years.

Or, be electrified daily.

Or, chew cinnamon daily.

Or, chew cinnamon daily, and swallow your spittle.

164. AN OLD STUBBORN PAIN IN THE BACK.

Steep root of water-fern, in water, till the water becomes thick aud clammy; then rub the parts therewith morning and evening.

Or, apply a plaster, and take, daily, balsam of copaiba.

Or, apply garlic and hog's lard to the feet. (Tried.)

165. THE PALSY.*

Be electrified, daily, for three months. from the places wherein the nerves spring. which are brought to the paralytic part. If the parts beneath the head are affected, the fault is in the spinal marrow: if half the body, half the marrow is touched.

---

* A palsy is the loss of motion or feeling, or both, in any particular part of the body.

A PALSEY may be cured in spring or summer, but rarely in winter.

Or, use the cold bath if you are under fifty, rubbing and sweating after it.

Or, shred white onions, and bake them gently in au earthen pot till they are soft; spread a thick plaster of this and apply it to the benumbed part, all over the side if need be. I have known this cure a person seventy-five years old.

Or, take tar-water morning and evening.

THIS helps all nervous disorders.

Or, take a tea-spoonful of powdered sage lying down in bed.

166. PALSY OF THE HANDS.

Wash them often in decoction of sage as hot as you can bear.

Or, boil a handful of elder-leaves, and two or three spoonsful of mustard-seed in a quart of water. Wash often in this as hot as may be.

167. PALSY OF THE MOUTH.

After purging well, chew mustard-seed often.

Or, gargle with juice of wood sage.

168. PALSY FROM WORKING WITH WHITE LEAD OR VERDIGRISE.

Use warm baths and a milk diet.

169. PALPITATION OR BEATING OF THE HEART.

Drink a pint of cold water.
Or, apply outwardly a rag dipped in vinegar.
Or, be electrified. (Tried.)
Or, take a decoction of mother-wort every night.

170. THE PILES, (TO PREVENT.)

Wash the parts daily with cold water.

171. THE PILES, (TO CURE.)

Apply warm treacle.
Or, a tobacco-leaf steeped in water twenty-four hours.
Or, a poultice of boiled brook-lime. It seldom fails.
Or, a bruised onion skinned, or roasted in ashes. It perfectly cures dry piles.
Or, varnish. It perfectly cures both the blind and bleeding piles. (Tried).
Or, fumigate with vinegar. wherein red hot flints have been quenched. This softens even scirrhus tumors.

172. THE INWARD PILES.

Swallow a pill of pitch fasting. One pill usually cures the bleeding piles.

Or, take twice a day, as much as lies on a shilling, of the thin skin of walnuts, powdered.

173. VIOLENT BLEEDING PILES.

Lightly boil the juice of nettles with a little sugar ; take two ounces. It seldom needs repeating.

174. THE PLAGUE, (TO PREVENT.)

Eat marigold flowers, daily, as a salad, with oil and vinegar.

Or, infuse rue, sage, mint, rosemary, wormwood, of each a handful, into two quarts of the sharpest vinegar, over warm embers for eight days : then strain it through a funnel, and add half an ounce of camphire dissolved in three ounces of rectified spitits of wine. With this wash the loins, face, and mouth, and snuff a little up the nose when you go abroad. Smell to a sponge dipped therein when you approach infected persons or places.

275. THE PLAGUE, [TO CURE.]

Cold water alone, drank largely, has cured it.

Or, an ounce or two of the juice of marigolds.

Or, after bleeding fifteen or sixteen ounces, drink very largely of water sharpened with spirit of vitriol.—*Dr. Dover.*

Or, a draught of brine as soon as seized: sweat in bed;
take no other drink for some hours.

Or, use lemon juice largely in every thing.

176. THE PLEURISY.

Take half a drachm of soot.

Or, take out the core of an apple, fill it up with white
frankincense, stop it close with the piece you cut out, and
roast it in ashes. Mash and eat it. [I.]

Or, a glass of tar-water warm every half hour.

Or, of decoction of nettles, and apply the boiled herb hot
as a poultice. I never knew it fail.

Or, a plaster of flour of brimstone and white of an egg.
(Tried.) This seldom fails.

In disordes of this kind Dr. Huxham advises: "Sip almost continually thin whey, barley-water, or hyssop tea,
sharpened with vinegar and water or lemon-juice. If the
spitting stop suddenly, take a gentle vomit. Likewise camphorated vinegar, with syrup of elder or raspberries, is
good." To appease the cough, take often, a little at a time,
of roasted apples, of strawberries, raspberries, or currants

177. TO ONE POISONED.

Give one or two grains of distilled verdigrise. It vomits
in an instant.

Let one poisoned by arsenicdissolve a quarter of an ounce

of salt of tartar in a pint of water, and drink every quarter of an hour as much as he can, till he is well.

Let one poisoned by opium take thirty drops of elixir of vitriol in cold water, every quarter of an hour, till the drowsiness or wildness ceases.

Or, a spoonful of lemon-juice.

Let one poisoned by mercury sublimate dissolve an ounce of salt of tartar in a gallon of water, and drink largely of it.

THIS will entirely destroy the force of the poison if it be used soon.

Nothing cures the African poison but a decoction of the roots of the sensitive plant

178. A POLYPUS IN THE NOSE.

Powder a lump of alum and snuff it up frequently : then dissolve powdered alum in brandy, dip lint therein, and apply it at going to bed.

179. A PRICK OR CUT THAT FESTERS.

Apply turpentine.

180. PTYALISM, OR CONTINUAL SPITTING.

A very violent and stubborn disorder of this kind was cured by chewing perpetually a little dry bread, and swallowing it with the spittle.

181. AN EASY PURGE.

Drink a pint of warmish water fasting, walking after it.

Or, a soft egg with a tea-spoonful of salt.

Or, infuse from half a drachm to two drachms of damask rose leaves, dried, in half a pint of warm water for twelve hours, and take it.

Or, infuse three drachms of senna, and a scruple of salt of tartar, in half a pint of river water for twelve hours; then strain and take it in the morning.

Wild ash is a plant of the very same nature with senna. Its leaves taken in double the quantity purge full as well and does not gripe as senna does.

The wild ash is called, in the north of England, round-tree, quick-beam, or wigan-tree. The leaves should be gathered when the tree is in flower.

182. A STRONGER PURGE.

Drink: half a pint of strong decoction of dock-root.

Or, the jalap powder in treacle, or any liquid in the morning fasting.

Or, the jalap powder may be made into pills.

Or, a table-spoonful of tincture of jalap in a morning, fasting, in a cup of cold camomile tea.

183. THE QUINSY*

Apply a large white bread toast half an inch thick, dip-

*Fever attended with difficulty of swallowing, and often of breathing.

ped in brandy, to the crown of the head till it dries.

Or, swallow slowly white rose-water mixed with syrup of mulberries. (Tried.)

Or, juice or jelly of black currants, or the decoction of the leaves or bark.

Or, draw in as hot as you can bear, for ten or twelve minutes together, the fumes of red-rose leaves, or camomile flowers, boiled in water and vinegar, or of a decoction of bruised hemp-seed.

This speedily cures the sore throat, peripneumony, and inflammation of the uvula.

184. A QUINSY OF THE BREAST *

Take from eight to twenty drops of laudanum lying down in bed. This helps.

Or, make an issue in the thigh. This cures.

185. THE RHEUMATISM.†

To prevent, wear washed wool under the feet.

To cure, use the cold bath with rubbing and sweating.

Or, apply warm steams.

Or, rub in warm treacle, and apply to the part brown pa-

---

* This is known by a sudden unaccountable pain and difficulty of breathing seizing a person in the night, or any violent motion.

† Rheumatical pains are generally most violent as soon as you are warm in bed : but there is a cold rheumatism which is most painful when the part is cold. Constant rubbing will cure this.

per smeared therewith ; change it in twelve hours. [Tried.]

Or, drink half a pint of tar-water morning and evening.

Or, steep six or seven cloves of garlic in half a pint of white wine ; drink it lying down. It sweats and frequently cures at once.

Or, mix flour of brimstone with honey, in equal quantities, take three teaspoonsful at night, two in the morning, and one afterwards, morning and evening, till cured. This succeeds oftener than any remedy I have found.

Or, live on new milk whey and white bread for fourteen days. This has cured one in a desperate case.

Or, pound the green stalks of English rhubarb in May or June, with an equal quantity of lump sugar. Take the quantity of a nutmeg of this three or four times a day. This seldom fails.

In a stubborn rheumatism, let your diet be barley-gruel, with currants, roasted apples, fresh whey, and light pudding.

186. TO RESTORE THE STRENGTH AFTER A RHEUMATISM.

Make a strong broth of cow-heels, and wash the parts with it warm twice a day. It has restored one who was quite a cripple, having no strength left either in his leg thigh, or loins.

Or, mix gum guaiacum in powder, with honey and treacle: take two or three tea-spoonsful [or as much as you can bear without purging], twice or thrice a day. This is the best medicine I have met with for the chronic rheumatism.

Or, dissolve one ounce of gum guaiacum in three ounces of spirits of wine : take sixty or eighty drops on loaf sugar, two or three times a day.   This is Dr. Hill's Essence of Bardana.

Or, drop thirty drops of volatile tincture of guaiacum on a lump of sugar. and take this in a glass of water every four hours.   It usually cures in a day.   (Tried.)

187. RICKETS, (to cure or prevent.)

Wash the child every morning in cold water.

188. RING WORMS.*

Apply rotten apples or pounded garlic.
Or, rub them with juice of house-leek.
Or, wash teem with Hungary water camphorated.
Or, twice a day with oil of sweet almonds and oil of tartar mixed.

189. RUNNING AT THE NOSE.

Snuff up a tea-spoonful of spirits of hartshorn

190. A RUPTURE.

Foment with hot aqua vitæ for two hours.

---

* Vulgarly called tetters.

Or, take agrimony, spleen-wort, Solomon's seal, straw-
berry roots, a handful of each ; pick and wash them well ;
stamp and boil them two hours in two quarts of white wine
in a vessel close stopped : strain and drink a large glass of
this every morning, and an hour after drink another. It
commonly cures in a fortnight. A good truss in the meantime is of great use, and perhaps the only thing to be de-
pended on.

"I place," says Dr. Riviere, "a broad plank sloping from
the side of the bed to the floor. On this I lay the patient
upon pillows, with his head downward. Then I foment the
part for half an hour with cloths, four times doubled, steeped
in cold water, gently touching it with my fingers. Afterwards I bind on it, many times doubled, a cloth shaped like
a triangle, wet in cold water. The gut is generally restored
to its place in a few hours. If not, I repeat the operation
twice a day, and in two or three days the disease is cured."

191. A RUPTURE IN CHILDREN.

Boil a spoonful of egg-shells dried in an oven, and powdered, in three quarters of a pint of milk. Feed the child
constantly with bread boiled in this milk.

192. A WINDY RUPTURE.

A poultice of the entrils of a cow on leather, strewing
some cummin seeds on it, and apply it hot. When cold put
on a new one. It commonly cures a child (keeping in bed)
in two days.

193. A SCALD HEAD.

Anoint it with Barbadoes tar.

Or, apply daily white wine vinegar.   (Tried.)

If wood soot is mixed with fresh butter into an ointment, and the head anointed with it every day it will generally cure it at the beginning ; but when it is become very bad, a a plaster should be made of gall, dried to the consistence of salve, and spread upon linen. This should be applied all over the parts affected, and continued on four or five days ; then it should be taken off and the head dressed with soot ointment as before.

After the cure, give two or three gentle purges.

If a proper regard was paid to cleanliness in the head and apparel of children, the scald head would seldom be seen.

194. THE SCIATICA.*

Is certainly cured by a purge taken in a few hours after it begins.

Or, use cold bathing and sweat, together with the flesh brush twice a day.

Or, boil nettles till soft : foment with the liquor, then apply the herb as a poultice. I have known this cure a sciatica of forty-five years standing.

Or, a mud made made of powdered pit coal and warm water. This frequently cures sores, weakness of the limbs,

---

* The sciatica is a violent pain in the hip, chiefly in the joints of the thigh bone.

most disorders of the legs, and swellings of the elbow joint, though accompanied with a fistula arising from a caries of the bone.

195. INFLAMMTION OR SWELLING OF THE SCROTUM.

Wash it thrice a day with a strong decoction of agrimony

196. A SCORBUTIC ATROPHY.*

Use cold bathing. Which also cures all scorbutic pains

197. SCORBUTIC GUMS.

Wash them daily with the decoction of the Peruvian bark, adding a little tincture of rosemary, with a solution of myrrh.

198. SCORBUTIC SORES.

A diet drink : Put half a pound of fresh-shaved lignum guaiacum [called by the blockmakers, lignum vitæ], and half an ounce of senna, into an earthen pot that holds six quarts. Add five quarts of soft water and lute the pot close

---

* Such a degree of the scurvy as causes the flesh to waste away like a consumption.

Set this in a kettle of cold water, and put it over a fire till it
has boiled three hours. Let it stand in the kettle till cold.
When it has stood one night, drink daily half a pint in new
milk warm, in the morning, fasting, and at four in the afternoon unless it purges too much, if so, take less. Wash with
a little of it. In three months all the sores will be dried up
(Tried).

199. SCURVY.†

Live on turnips for a month.

Or, take tar water, morning and evening, for three months.

Or, three spoonsful of nettle juice every morning.
(Tried.)

*Or, decoction of burdock. Boil three ounces of the
dried root in two quarts of water to three pints. Take a
half pint daily. A decoction of the leaves (boiling one leaf
four minutes in a quart of water,) has the same effect.

Or, take a cupful of the juice of goose grass in a morning
fasting, for a month ; it is frequently called hariff, or cleav-
ers, I have known many persons cured by it.

Or, pound into a pulp, of Seville orangers, sliced, rind and
all, and powder sugar, equal quantities. Take a tea-spoonful three or four times a day. (Tried.)

Or, squeeze the juice of half a Seville orang into a pint of

---

† The scurvy is known by heaviness of the body, weariness, rottenness
of the gums, and yellow, lead, or violet colored spots on the legs or
arms.

N. B. A scurvy attended with costiveness (which is the most common)
is termed a hot scurvy, one attended with looseness, a cold scurvy.

milk over the fire. Sweeten the whey with loaf sugar, and drink it every morning new milk warm. To make any whey, milk should be skimmed after it is boiled.

Or, pour three quarts of boiling water on a quart of ground malt; stir them well, and let the mixture stand close covered for four hours; strain it off and use this as common drink : in hot weather, brew this fresh every day. It will hardly fail.

Or, take morning and evening a spoonful or two of lemon juice and sugar. It is a precious remedy, and well tried.— *Dr. Macbridge.*

Water and and garden cresses, mustard, and juice of scurvy grass help in a cold scurvy.

When there is a continual salt taste in the mouth, take a pint of lime-water morning and evening.

200. A BROKEN SHIN.

Bind a dry oak leaf upon it.

Or, put on a bit of white paper moistened with spittle. It will stay on till the place is well. (Tried.) This cures a cut.

201. SHINGLES.*

Drink sea water every morning for a week : towards the close bathe also.

Or, apply pounded garlic.

---

* A kind of ring worm which encircles the body like a belt of a hand's breadth.

202. SICKISHNESS IN THE MORNING.

Eat nothing after six in the evening.
 Or, drink   half a pint of water impregnated with fixed
air.

203. SINEWS SHRUNK.

Rub the part every morning with fasting spittle.
Or, beat the yolk of a new-laid egg, mix it with a spoonful of water, and rub the part with it before the fire three or
four times a day.

204. SKIN RUBBED OFF.

Apply pounded all-heal. It seldom needs repeating.
Ɔr, a bit of white paper with spittle.

205. SMALL POX.

Drink largely of toast and water.
Or, let your whole food be milk and water, mixed with a
little white bread.
 Or, milk and apples.
Take good care to have free, pure and cool air.
Therefore open the casement every day ; only do not let it
chill the patient
If they strike in, and convulsions follow, drink a pint of
cold water immediately. This instantly stops the convulsion,
and drives out the poek. (Tried.)

There may be pustules a second time, coming out and ripening like the small pox, but it is bareiy a cutaneous disorder.

" In violent cases, bleed in the foot ; bathe the legs in warm water twice or thrice a day, before and at the eruption, and apply boiled turnips to the feet. Never keep the head too hot.

" In very low depressed cases wine may be given, and if the pustules lie buried in the skin, a gentle vomit ; in many cases a gentle purge of manna, cream of tartar or rhubarb.

"In the Crude Ichorose small pox, a dish of coffee now and then, with a little thick milk in it, has often quieted the vexatious cough.

" After the incrustation is formed, change the sick, but let it be with very dry warm linen.—*Dr. Huxham.*

206. A LONG RUNNING SORE IN THE BACK.

Was entirely cured by eating betony in everything.

Or, take every morning two or three spoonsful of nettle juice, and apply nettles bruised in a mortar to the part. This cures any old sore or ulcer. (I.)

207. A SORE LEG.

Bind a diculum plaster, an inch broad, round the leg, just above the sore, and foment it morning and evening with hot water.

Any sore is healed by a plaster of mutton-suet, even though it fester or breed proud flesh.

208. A SORE MOUTH.

Apply the white of an egg beat up with loaf sugar.

Or, gargle with the juice of cinquefoil.

Or, boil together a pound of treacle, three yolks of eggs, an ounce of bole amoniac, and the quantity of a nutmeg of alum a quarter of an hour. Apply this to the sore part, or to an aching tooth. (Tried.)

209. A SORE THROAT.

Take a pint of cold water lying down in bed. (Tried.)

Or, apply a chin-stay of roasted figs.

Or, a flannel sprinkled with spirits of hartshorn to the throat, rubbing Hungary water on the top of the head. (Tried.)

Or, snuff a little honey up the nose.

An old sore throat was cured by living wholly on apples and apple-water.

210. AN INFLAMED SORE THROAT.

Lay nitre and loaf sugar, mixed, on the tongue.

211. A PUTRID SORE THROAT.

Lay on the tongue a lump of sugar dipped in brandy.

212. A SPRAIN.

Hold the part in very cold water for two hours. (Tried.)
Or, apply cloths dipped therein, four times doubled, for two hours, changing them as they grow warm.

Or, bathe it in good crab verjuice.

Or, boil bran in wine vinegar to a poultice. Apply this warm and renew it once in twelve hours.

Weakness remaining afrer a sprain, is cured by fomenting the part daily with beef-brine.

Suppose the ancle sprained : 1st. Foment it with warm vinegar four or five times every four hours. 2nd. Stand, if you can, three or four minutes at a time on both your feet, and frequently move the sprained foot. Sometimes also while sitting with your foot on a low stool, move it to and fro. 3rd. Let it be gently rubbed with a warm hand at least thrice a day. 4. Two hours after every application of the vinegar, let it be just wetted with spirits of wine and then gently rubbed.

213. A VENOMOUS STING.

Apply the juice of honey-suckle leaves.

Or, a poultice of bruised plantain and honey.

Or, take inwardly, one drachm of black currant leaves powdered. It is an excellent counter-poison.

214. THE STING OF A BEE.

Apply honey.

Or, mix a little turpentine with flour in the yolk of an egg, and apply it as a plaster. This cures in a desperate case.

215, THE STING OF A NETTLE.

Rub the part with the juice of nettles.

216. THE STING OF A WASP.

Rub the part with the bruised leaves of house-leek, water-cresses or rue.

Or, apply treacle or sweet oil.

Or, bruised onions or garlic.

217. STING OF BEE OR WASP IN THE EYE.

Apply carduus bruised with the white of an egg, renew it if it grows dry.

218. STING IN THE GULLET.

Beat well together, with a spoon, some honey and sweet oil with a little vinegar ; swallow a spoonful every minute till ease is procured.

219. A STITCH IN THE SIDE.

Apply treacle spread on hot toast. (Tried.)

220. ACCIDENTAL SICKISHNESS, OR PAIN IN THE STOMACH.

Vomit with a quart of warm water. Do this twice or thrice, omiting a day between.

221. PAIN IN THE STOMACH FROM BAD DIGESTION.

Take fasting, or in the fit, half a pint of camomile tea. Do this five or six mornings.

Or, drink the juice of half a large lemon, or sweet orange, immediately after dinner every day.

Or, in the fit a glass of vinegar.

Or, take two or three tea spoonsful of stomachic tincture in a glass of water, thrice a day.

THE tincture is made thus : Gentian root, sliced, one ounce ; orange peel, dried, half an ounce ; cochineal, fifteen grains ; proof brandy one pint : in three or four days it is fit for use. This is useful in all disorders that arise from a relaxed stomach.

222. CHOLERIC PAINS IN THE STOMACH.

Take half a pint of decoction of ground-ivy, with a tea-spoonful of the powder of it, five or six mornings. (I.)

223. COLDNESS IN THE STOMACH.

Take a spoonful of the syrup of the juice of carduus benedictus, fasting, for three or four mornings. (I.)

Or, chew a leaf of carduus every morning, and swallow the spittle. (Tried).

224. PAIN IN THE STOMACH, WITH COLDNESS AND WIND.

Swallow five or six corns of pepper for six or seven mornings. (Tried.)

225. STONE, (TO PREVENT.)

Eat a small crust of bread every morning. (Tried).

Or, drink a pint of warm water, daily, just before dinner. After discharging one stone, this will prevent the generating of another. Stoop down and raise up again. If you feel pain as if cut through the middle, the pain is not from the stone, but rheumatism. Beware of costiveness. Use no violent diuretics. Mead is a proper drink.

Or, slice a large onion, pour half a pint of warm water upon it. After it has stood twelve hours, drink the water. Do this every morning till you are well.

226. IN A RAGING FIT.

* Beat onions into a pulp and apply them as a poultice to the back, or to the groin.   It gives speedy ease in the most racking pain.   (Tried.)

227. STONE, (to ease or cure.)

Boil half a pound of parsnips in a quart of water.   Drink a glass of this morning and evening, and use no other drink all the day.   It usually cures in six weeks.

Or, take morning and evening a tea-spoonful of onions, calcined in a fire shovel into white ashes, in white wine.   An ounce will often dissolve the stone.

Or, take a tea-spoonful of violet seed, powdered, morning and evening.   It both wastes the stone and brings it away.

Or, drink largely of water impregnated with fixed air.

Those who have not a convenient apparatus, may substitute the following method : Dissolve sixteen grains of salt of tartar in six spoonsful of water, to which add as much water aciduated with oil of vitriol as will neutralize the salt. They are to be gradually mixed with each other, so as to prevent the efferescence or dissipation of the fixed air as much as possible.

228. STONE IN THE KIDNEYS.

Use the cold bath.

Or, drink half a pint of water every morning.

Or, boil an ounce of common thistle-root, and four

drachms of liquorice, in a pint of water.   Drink of it every morning.

229. STOPPAGE IN THE KIDNEYS.

Take decoction, or juice, or syrup of ground-ivy, morning and evening.

Or, half a pint of tar-water.

Or, twelve grains of salt of amber in a little water.

230. THE STRANGUARY.

Sit over the steam of warm water.

Or, drink largely of decoction of turnips, sweetened with clarified honey.

* Or, of warm lemonade.   (Tried.)

Or, dissolve half an ounce of saltpeter in a quart of water. Drink a glass of it every hour.

231. SUNBURN, (SMARTING.)

Wash the face with sage tea.

232. A FRESH SURFEIT.

Take about the size of a nutmeg of the green tops of wormwood.

233. TO STOP PROFUSE SWEATING.

Drink largely of cold water.

234. TO PREVENT IT.

Mix an ounce of tincture of Peruvian bark with half an ounce of spirit of vitriol. Use a tea-spoonful morning and evening in a glass of water.

235. TO CURE NIGHT SWEATS.

Drink a gill of warm milk at lying down.

236. SWELLED GLANDS IN THE NECK.

Take sea-water every other day.

237. INDOLENT SWELLINGS

Are often cured by warm sweats.

238. SOFT AND FLABBY SWELLINGS.

Pump cold water on them daily.
Or, use constant friction.
Or, proper bandages.

239. WHITE SWELLING IN THE JOINTS.

Hold the part half an hour every morning under a pump

or cock.   This cures all pains in the joints.   It seldom fails.
(Tried.)

Or, pour on it daily a stream of warm water.

Or, a stream of cold water one day, and warm the next,
and so on, by turns.

Use these remedies at first, if possible.   It is likewise
proper to intermix gentle purges to prevent a relapse.

Or, boiled nettles.

240. TO DISSOLVE WHITE OR HARD SWELL-
INGS.

Take white roses, elder flowers, leaves of fox-gloves, and
and of St. John's wort, a handful   of each ; mix with hog's
lard and make an ointment.

Or, hold them morning and evening in the steam of vinegar poured on red hot flints.

241. TO FASTEN THE TEETH.

Put powdered alum, the quantity of a nutmeg, in a quart
of spring water for twenty-four hours : then strain the water
and gargle with it.

Or, gargle often with phyllera leaves boiled with a little
alum in forge water.

242. TO CLEAN THE TEETH.

Rub them with ashes of burned bread.

243. TO PREVENT THE TOOTH-ACHE.

Wash the mouth with cold water every morning, and rince them after every meal.

Or, rub the teeth often with tobacco ashes.

244. TO CURE THE TOOTH-ACHE.

Be electrified through the teeth.   (Tried.)

Or, apply to the aching tooth an artificial magnet.

Or, rub the cheek a quarter of an hour.

Or, lay roasted parings of turnips, as hot as may be, behind the ear.

Or, put a leaf of betony, up the nose.

Or, lay bruised or boiled nettles to the cheek.   (Tried.)

Or, lay a clove of garlic on the tooth.

Or, hold a slice of apple lightly boiled between the teeth. (Tried.)

Or, keep the feet in warm water, and rub them well with bran just before bed time.   (Tried.)

THE first twenty teeth generally last till the sixth or seventh year ; after that, till the fourteenth or fifteenth year ; they fall out one by one, and are succeeded by others.

The shedding of teeth is wisely intended, and brought about in a singular manner.   Their hardness will not admit of distension like other parts of the body.   Hence, after an enlargement of the jaw-bone, the original teeth are no longer able to fill up the cavities of it.   They must stand unsupported by each other, and leave spaces between them.

Under the first teeth, therefore, is placed a new set, which,
by constant pressing upon their roots, rob them of their
nourishment, and finally push them out of their sockets.

245. TOOTH-ACHE FROM COLD AIR.

Keep the mouth full of warm water.

246. TEETH SET ON EDGE.

Rub the tops of the teeth with a dry towel.
There is no such thing as worms in the teeth.   Children's
using coral is always useless, often hurtful.

" Forcing the teeth into order is always dangerous.   Fill
ing is generally hurtful.

"All rough and cutting powders destroy the teeth, so do all
common tinctures.

" Sweet meats are apt to hurt the teeth, if the mouth be
not rinsed after them.   Cracking nuts often breaks off the
enamel ; so does biting thread in two.

" Constant use of tooth-picks is a bad practice, constant
smoking of tobacco destroys many good sets of teeth."–*Dr.
Beardmore.*

247. EXTREME THIRST, [WITHOUT A FEVER.]

Drink spring water in which a little sal prunello is dissolved.

248. PAIN IN THE TESTICLES.

Apply pellitory of the wall beaten up into a poultice changing morning and evening.

249. TESTICLES INFLAMED.

Boil bean flower in three parts of water, one part vinegar.

250. TO DRAW OUT THORNS, SPLINTERS, AND BONES.

Apply nettle-roots and salt.
Or, turpentine spread on leather.

251. THRUSH.*

Mix juice of calendine with honey to the thickness of cream. Infuse a little powdered saffron, let this simmer a while and scum it; apply it where needed with a feather. At the same time give eight or ten grains of rhubarb; to grown persons twenty.

Or, take an ounce of clarified honey, having scummed off all the dross from it, put in a drachm of roche-alum finely powdered, and stir them well together. Let the child's mouth be rubbed well with this five or six times a day, with

---

* Little white ulcers in the mouth.

a bit of rag tied upon the end of a stick ; and though it be the thorough thrush, it will cure it in a few days. I never knew it fail.

Or, burn scarlet cloth to ashes and blow them into the mouth. This seldom fails.

252. TONSILS SWELLED.

Wash them well with lavender-water.

253. TORPOR OR NUMBNESS OF THE LIMBS.

Use the cold bath with rubbing and sweating.

255. TYMPANY OR WINDY DROPSY.

Use the cold bath with purges intermixed.

Or, mix juice of leeks and of elder. Take two or three spoonsful of this morning and evening. (Tried.)

Or, eat a few parched peas every hour.

256. A VEIN OR SINEW CUT.

Apply the inner green rind of hazel, fresh scraped.

257. THE VERTIGO, OR SWIMMING IN THE HEAD.

Take a vomit or two.

Or, use the cold bath for a month.

Or, in a May morning about sun-rise snuff up the dew, daily, that is on mallow leaves.

Or, apply to the top of the head, shaven, a plaster of flour of brimstone and white of eggs. (Tried.)

Or, take every morning half a drachm of mustard-seed.

Or, mix one part of salt of tartar with three parts of cream of tartar; take a tea-spoonful in a glass of water, every morning, fasting. This is serviceable when the vertigo springs from acid, tough phlegm in the stomach.

258. VIGILIA, OR INABILITY TO SLEEP.

Apply to the forehead, for two hours, cloths four times doubled, dipped in cold water. I have known this applied to a lying-in woman and her life saved thereby.

Or, take a grain or two of camphire. It is both safer and surer than opium.

Assafœtida, from ten to thirty grains, likewise will in most cases have as much effect as opium. Drink no green tea in the afternoon.

259. BITE OF A VIPER OR RATTLE SNAKE.

Apply bruised garlick.

Or, rub the place immediately with common oil. Query, would not the same cure the bite of a mad dog? Would it not be worth while to make a trial on a mad dog?

260. TO PREVENT THE BITE OF A VIPER

Rub the hands with the juice of radishes.

261. AN ULCER.

Dry and powder a walnut leaf and strew it . on, and lay another walnut leaf on that. (Tried.)

Or, boil walnut tree leaves in water with a little sugar. Apply a cloth dipped in this, changing it once in two days. This has done wonders.

Or, foment morning and evening with a decoction of walnut-tree leaves on. This has cured foul bones ; yea, and a leprosy. (Tried.)

262. ULCER IN THE BLADDER OR KIDNEYS.

Take a decoction of agrimony thrice a day.
Or, decoction, powder, or syrup of horsetail.

263. ULCER IN THE GUM OR JAW.

Apply honey of roses sharpened with spirits of vitriol.

Or, fill the whites of eggs boiled hard and slit, with myrrh and sugar-candy, powdered. Tie them up, and hang them on sticks lying across a glass. A liquid distils, with which anoint the sores often in a day.

264. A FISTULOUS ULCER.

Apply wood-beteny, bruised, changing it daily.

265. A BLEEDING VARICOUS ULCER IN THE LEG.

Was cured by constant cold bathing.

266. A MALIGNANT ULCER.

Foment, morning and evening, with a decoction of mint ; then sprinkle on it finely powdered rue.

Or, burn to ashes, but not too long, the gross stalks on which the red coleworts grow. Make a plaster with fresh butter. Change it once a day.

Or, apply a poultice of boiled parsnips. This will cure even when the bone is foul.

Or, be electrified. (Tried.)

267. AN ULCER IN THE URETHRA*

Take a clove of garlic morning and evening.

---

* The urethra is the passage of the urine.

268. AN EASY AND SAFE VOMIT.

Pour a dish of tea on twenty grains of ipecacuanha. You may sweeten it if you please. When it has stood four or five minutes, pour the tea clear off and drink it.

269. TO STOP VOMITING.

Apply a large onion, slit across the grain, to the pit of the stomach. (Tried.)

Or, take a spoonful of lemon juice and six grains of salt of tartar.

270. BLOODY URINE.

Take twice a day a pint of decoction of agrimony.

Or, of decoction of yarrow.

271. URINE BY DROPS, WITH HEAT AND PAIN.

Drink nothing but lemonade. (Tried)

Or, beat up the pulp of five or six roasted apples with a quart of water. Use it at lying down. It commonly cures before morning.

272. INVOLUNTARY URINE.

Use the cold bath.

Or, take a tea-spoonful of powdered agrimony in a little water morning and evening.

Or, a quarter of a pint of alum posset drink every night.

Or, foment with rose leaves and plantain leaves, boiled in smith's forge water ; then apply plasters of alum and bole armoniac made up with oil and vinegar.

Or, apply a blister to the os-sacrum. It seldom fails.

273. SHARP URINE.

Take two spoonsful of fresh juice of ground-ivy.

274. SUPPRESSION OF URINE.

Sometimes relieved by bleeding

Or, drink largely of warm lemonade.

Or, a scruple of nitre every two hours.

Or, take a spoonful of the juice of lemon sweetened with syrup of violets.

Or, seven grains of mercurius dulcis.

275. UVULA INFLAMED.*

Gargle with a decoction of beaten hemp-seed.

Or, with a decoction of dandelion.

Or, touch it frequently with camphorated spirits of wine·

---

* This is usually called the palate of the mouth.

276. UVULA RELAXED.

Bruise the veins of a cabbage leaf and lay it hot on the crown of the head ; repeat, if needed, in two hours. I never knew it fail.

Or. gargle with an infusion of mustard-seed.

277. WARTS.

Rub them daily with a radish.

Or, water in which sal amoniac is dissolved.

Or, with juice of marigold flowers : it will hardly fail.

Qr, apply bruised purslain as a poultice, changing it twice a day. It cures in seven or eight days.

278. WEAKNESS IN THE ANCLES.

Hold them in cold water a quarter of an hour morning and evening.

279. A SOFT WEN.

Wrap leaves of sorrel in a wet paper, and roast them in the embers : mix it with finely sifted ashes into a poultice. Apply this warm, daily.

Dr. Reviere says : "I cured a wen as big as a large fist thus : I made an instrument of hard wood, like the stone with which the painters grind their colors on a marble.

With this I rubbed it half an hour twice a day; then I laid on a suppurating plaster very hot, which I kept on four or five days. The wen suppurated and was opened. Afterwards all the substance turned into matter, and was evacuated. Thus I have cured many since.

280. THE WHITES.

Live chastely; feed sparringly; use exercise constantly; sleep moderately, but never lying on your back.

Take eight grains of jalap every eight days. This usually cures in five weeks.

Or, first bleed; then purge thrice with twenty grains of rhubarb, and five of calomel.

Or, boil four or five leaves of the white holly-hock in a pint of milk with a little sugar, then add a tea-spoonful of balm of Gilead. Drink this every morning. It rarely fails.

Or, make Venice turpentine, flour, and fine sugar, equal quantities, into small pills. Take three or four of these morning and evening. This also cures most pains in the back.

Or, take yellow resin, powdered, one ounce; conserve of roses, half an ounce; powdered rhubarb, three drachms; syrup a sufficient quantity to make an electuary. Take a large tea-spoonful of this twice a day, in a cup of confrey-root tea.

Or, in a quarter of a pint of water, wherein three drachms of tamarinds and a drachm of lentisk-wood has been boiled. When cold, infuse senna, one drachm; coriander-seed and liquorice, a drachm and a half each. Let them stand all night.   Strain the liquor in the morning, and drink it daily two hours before breakfast.

281.   A WHITLOW.

Apply treacle.   (Tried.)
Or, honey and flour.   (Tried.)
Or, a poultice of chewed bread.   Shift it once a day.
Or, a poultice of powdered pit coal and warm water.

*282.   WORMS.

Use two tea-spoonsful of brandy, sweetened with loaf sugar, every morning.

Or, a spoonful of the juice of lemons.

Or, two spoonsful of nettle juice.

Or, boil four ounces of quicksilver an hour in a quart of clear water :   pour it off and bottle it up.   You may use the same quicksilver again and again.   Use this for common drink ; or at least, night and morning for a week or two. Then purge off the dead worms with fifteen or twenty grains of jalap.

Or, take two tea-spoonsful of worm seed mixed with treacle, for six mornings.

---

* A child may be known to have the worms by chilliness, paleness, hollow eyes, itching of the nose, starting in sleep, and an unusual stinking breath.   Worms are never found in children that live wholly on milk.

Or, one, two, or three drachms of powdered fern-root
boiled in mead. This kills both the flat and round worms.
Repeat the medicine from time to time.

Or give one tea-spoonful of syrup of bear's foot at bed
time, and one or two in the morning, for two or three suc-
cessive days, to children between two and six years of age,
regulating the dose according to the strength of the patient.

Syrup of bear's foot is made thus : Sprinkle the green
leaves with vinegar, stamp and strain out the juice, and add
to it a sucfficient quantity of coarse sugar. This is the
most powerful medicine for long round worms.

Bruising the green leaves of bear's foot and smelling often
at them, sometimes expels worms.

Or, boil half an ounce of aloes, powdered, with a few
sprigs of rue, wormwood, and camomile, in a half a pint
of gall, to the consistency of a plaster ; spread this on thin
lether and apply it to the stomach, changing it every twelve
hours, for three days ; then take fifteen grains of jalap, and
it will bring vast quantities of worms away, some burst, and
some alive. This will cure when no internal medicine avails.

283. FLAT WORMS.

Mix a tablespoonful of Norway tar in a pint of small beer ;
take it as you can in the morning, fasting. This brought
away a tape worm thirty-six feet in length.

Or take from two to five grains of gamboge made into
a bolus, in the morning, fasting, drinking after it a little
weak green tea, and likewise when it begins to operate, till
the worm is evacueted. The dose must be regulated accord-

ing to the patient's strength ; for neither this nor any other medicine given as an alterative, is of the least service in this disorder. If the head of the worm be fixed in the upper orfice of the stomach, a smart shock from the electrifying machine will probably dislodge it : then purge. To prevent —avoid drinking stagnated water.

284. WOUNDS.

If you have not an honest surgeon at hand
Apply juice or powder of yarrow—(I.)
Or, bind leaves of ground-ivy upon it.
Or, wood-betony bruised. It quickly heals even cut veins and sinews, and drawsout thorns or splinters.
Or. keep the part in cold water for an hour, keeping the wounds closed with your thumb ; then bind on the thin skin of an egg-shell for days or weeks, till it falls off itself. Regard not though it prick or shoot for a time.

285 INWARD WOUNDS.

Infuse yarrow twelve hours in warm water. Use a cup of this four times a day.

286. PUTRID WOUNDS.

Wash them morning and evening with warm decoction of agrimony. If they heal too soon, and a matter gathers underneath, apply a poultice of the leaves pounded, changing them once a day till well.

Or, apply a carrot poultice ; but if the gangrene comes on, apply a wheat poultice (after it has been by the fire till it begins to ferment) nearly cold. It will not fail.

287. WOUNDED TENDONS.

Boil comfrey roots to a thick mucilage or jelly, and apply this as a poultice, changing it twice a day.

288. TO OPEN A WOUND THAT IS CLOSED TO SOON.

Apply bruised centuary.

MEDICINES.

DAFFY'S ELIXIR.

Take of the best senna, guaiacum, liquorice sliced small, aniseeds, coriander seeds, and elecampane-root, of each half an ounce ; raisins of the sun,* stoned, a quarter of a pound : let them all be bruised and put into a quart of the best brandy. Let it stand by the fire a few days. and then strain it.

ANOTHER RECEIPT FOR DAFFY'S ELIXIR.

Take of senna leaves, two ounces † coriander-seeds, a quarter of an ounce ; proof spirit, or brandy, three pints : put all the ingredients into a bottle for four or five days, shaking it frequently ; strain off the tincture, and add three ounces of powdered sugar candy. This medicine is more active than the preceding, and is calculated to remove obstructions in the bowels, in cholics and other complaints that require purging, especially when castor oil has not had the

---

* Sun cured.   † Jalap one ounce.

desired effect.   The dose is one, two, or three table-spoonsful, in a cup of camomile tea, or water.

TURLINGTON'S BALSAM.

Take balsams of Peru and Tolu, of each half an ounce ;
gum storax, in tears, and gum guaiacum, of each one ounce ;
gum benjamin, an ounce and a half ; hepatic aloes and frankincense, of each two drachms : let the gum be bruised, and
put all the ingredients into a quart of rectified spirits of
wine ; shake the bottle frequently, and in eight days it is fit
for use.

This is indeed a most excellent medicine for man or beast,
or for any fresh wound.   I know none like it.

SCOTCH PILLS.

Dissolve two ounces of hepatic aloes, with a small spoonful of sweet oil and as much water, in a porringer over a
small fire.   When it is of a proper consistence, make it into
pills with or without liquorice powder.

EMETIC TARTAR VOMIT.

Dissolve four grains of emetic tartar in half a pint of hot
water ; stir it about well : when it is cold it is fit for use.
Take two table-spoonsful every quarter of an hour till it
operates ; after which no more of the vomit must be taken.
Drink a small cup of gruel, or weak camomile tea after every

puke to work it off. A pint or a pint and a half of gruel of tea is generally sufficient. To settle the stomach, drink a little weak brandy and water, and lie down half an hour.

One table-spoonful of the emetic tartar water, every quarter of an hour till it pukes, is sufficient for weak people; while others again require four times as much. A child of a month old may take a small tea-spoonful every quarter of an hour ; one of three months old will require two tea-spoonful, and so in proportion to their age and strength. Children require nothing to work off a vomit ; and a pint or a pint and a half of gruel or camomile tea is sufficient for adults. It is an absurd and pernicious practice to drink pint after pint of hot liquids to work off a vomit, and frequently leaves a very great relaxation of the stomach, which does not recover its tone for some months afterwards.

The design of giving a vomit in the manner above described, is in order that it may work in the gentlest manner possible. If it operates two, or three, or four times, it is sufficient. Violent vomits are often attended with dangerous consequences; whereas gentle ones may be repeated two or three times a week if necessary.

If a vomit works too violently, drink moderately of weak brandy and water, and apply a raw onion cut in two to the pit of the stomach.

The best time for taking a vomit is in a morning, fasting. But in cases where no time is to be lost, it may be taken at eleven o'clock, or in the evening.

Persons who are costive, should not venture upon a vomit till the costiveness is removed, which must be done in an hour or two's time by a clyster, or a small dose of jalap powder, or any other opening medicine.

In consumptive cases, and in the dysentery cases, ipeca-cuanha is the proper vomit. The emetic tartar is best cal-culated for- removing acidity, bile, and putrid matter from the stomach. In the beginning of some nervous and putrid fevers, where the pulse is weak, and the stomach loaded with sour, fœtid, yellow or green matter, there is perhaps no medi-cine equal to it. The heaviness, listlessness, pain in the loins, and head-ache, are generally removed before morn-ing.

Emetic tartar, when it is prescribed with judgment and taken properly, is one of the hest medicines known at this day. I have given it to many thousand patients with the utmost safety, and with the greatest advantage. I prefer it in every case to Jame's fever powder, though a medium com-posed of the same materials. The operations of emetic tar-tar may be directed to the stomach, the bowels, or the skin, as the case requires.

Some of the quack doctors mix powdered ginger with the emetic tartar, and call it the ginger vomit. I do not know that this is any injury to the medicine ; but some of the low country druggists adulterate it with chalk or magnesia : these articles are only hurtful by preventing the purchasers knowing exactly the quantity they ought to take. It is, there-fore, necessary to apply to apothecaries or druggists on whose veracity you can depend.

AN EXCELLENT EYE-WATER.

Take flowers of zinc and white copperas, of each a quar-ter of an ounce, water half a pint ; mix them together. It is used in the same manner as the white copperas eye-water but in most cases is greatly prefferable, particularly in the inflammation of the-lids, and any external or internal excorciation.   If it is too sharp, add a little more water to it.

COLD BATHING†

CURES YOUNG CHILDREN OF

Convulsions*	Inflammation of the ears
Coughs	navel, and mouth
Cutaneous inflammations,	Rickets
pimples, and scabs	Suppression of urine
Gravel	Vomiting
	Want of sleep

IT PREVENTS GROWTH OF HEREDITARY

Apoplexies	King's Evil
Asthmas	Melancholy
Blindness	Palsies
Consumptions	Rheumatism
Deafness	Stone
Gout	

---

* And this I apprehend accounts for its frequently curing the bite of a mad dog, especially if it be repeated for twenty-five or thirty days successively.

† Persons of feeble constitution should use it with care, and not remain too long in the bath; after the bath, rub the body until there is a glow over the whole surface.

Yet by this note let no one discontinue the use of baths, for they are approved by all when used properly.

WATER DRINKING

GENERALLY PREVENTS

Apoplexies
Asthmas
Convulsions
Gout
Hysteric fits

Madness
Palsies
Stone
Trembling.

To this children should be used from their cradles.

The best water to drink, especially for those who are much troubled with the wind, is rain water. After it has settled, draw it off clear into another vessel and it will keep sweet for a long time.

ELECTRIFYING

IN A PROPER MANNER, CURES

St. Anthony's Fire
Blindness
Blood extravasated
Bronchocele
Burns or scalds
Coldness in the feet
Contraction of the limbs
Convulsions
Cramp
Deafness
Falling sickness
Feet violently disordered
Felons
Fistula Lachrymalis
Fits

Lock jaws and joints
Leprosy
Menstrual obstruction
Opthalmia
Pain in the stomach
Palsy
Palpitation of the heart
Restores bulk and fulness to
    wasted limbs
Rheumatism
Ring worms
Sciatica
Shingles
Sinews shrunk
Spasm

Flooding
Ganglions
Gout
Head-ache
Imposthumes
Inflammation
Involuntary motion of the eye-lids
King's evil
Knots in the flesh
Lameness

Stiff joints
Sprains, however old
Surfeit
Swellings of all sorts
Sore throat
Tooth-ache
Ulcers
Wens
Wasting
Weakness of the legs

Nor have I yet known one single instance wherein it has done harm ; so that I cannot but doubt the the veracity of those who have affirmed the contrary. Dr. De Haen positively affirms it can do no hurt in any case ; that is, unless the shock be immoderately strong.

The best method is to give fifty, or even a hundred small shocks each time; but let them be so gentle as not terrify the patient in the least.

Drawing sparks removes those tumors on the eye-lids, called barley-corns, by exciting local inflammation, and promoting suppuration.

FASTING SPITTLE

OUTWARDLY APPLIED EVERY MORNING HAS SOMETIMES RE-

LIEVED AND SOMETIMES CURED

Blindness
Contracted sinews from a cut
Cuts (fresh)

Corns (mixed with chewed bread and applied every morning
Deafness

Eyelids red and inflamed
Scorbutic tetters

Sore legs
Warts

TAKEN INWARDLY IT RELIEVES OR CURES

Asthmas
Cancers
Falling sickness
Gout
Gravel
King's evil

Leprosy
Palsy
Rheumatism
Swelled liver
Stone
Scurvy

The best way is to eat about an ounce of hard bread, or sea-biscuit, every morning, fasting, two or three hours after. This should be done, in stubborn cases, for a month or six weeks.

NERVOUS AND PARALYTIC

DISORDERS ARE FREQUENTLY CURED BY THE COLD BATH,
BUT PARTICULARLY

Asthma
Agues of every sort
Atrophy
Blindness*
Cancer
Chin Cough
Coagulated blood after
    bruises
Consumptions
Convulsions
Coughs
Complication of distempers
Convulsive pains*
Deafness
Dropsy

Fevers (violent)
Gout (running)
Hectic Fevers
Hysteric pains*
Incubus
Inflammations*
Involuntary stool or urine*
Lameness
Leprosy (old)
Lethargy
Loss of appetite,* smell,*
    speech,* taste
Nephritic pains
Palpitation of the heart
Stone in the kidneys

Pains in the back, joints, stomach
Rheumatism
Rickets
Rupture
Suffocations
Surfeits (at the beginning)
Sciatica*
Scorbutic pains*
Swelling on the joints
Epilepsy

Torpor of the limbs, even when the use of them is lost
Tetanus
Tympany
Vertigo
St. Vitus' dance
Vigilia
Varicose ulcers
Whites

But in all cases where the nerves are obstructed, such as those marked thus* you should go to bed immediately after and sweat.

'Tis often necessary to use the hot bath a few days before you use the cold.

Wise parents should dip their children in cold water every morning, till they are three-quarters old ; and afterwards the hands and feet.

Washing the head every morning in cold water prevents rheums, and cures coughs, old head-aches, and sore eyes.

MANNER OF MAKING PILLS.—Use syrup or the best castile soap to soften the medicines ; and to thicken them, use pulverised licorice-root sufficient to give the proper consist_ ency. When made, dust the pills with the licorice powder. —ED.

VINEGAR AND LEMON-JUICE vapor diffused through the rooms of the sick, is both agreeable and wholesome.—ED.

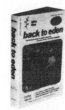
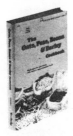
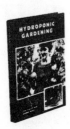
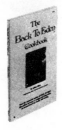